SOFTBILLS

SOFTBILLS
Care, Breeding and Conservation

Martin Vince

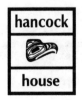
hancock house

ISBN 0-88839-393-8
Copyright © 1996 Martin Vince

Cataloging in Publication Data
Vince, Martin, 1964-
 Softbills

 ISBN 0-88839-393-8

 1. Softbills. I. Title.
 SF473.S64V55 1996   636.6'8   C96-910396-4

All rights reserved. No part of this publication may be reproduced, stored in a retrieval system or transmitted, in any form or by any means, electronic, mechanical, photocopying, recording, or otherwise, without the prior written permission of Hancock House Publishers.
Printed in Hong Kong

Production: Lorna Brown
Editing: Nancy Miller
Author photo: Renata Tramontana-Vince
Cover photos: David and Laurel Hancock
  Upper left: Red-crested touraco, *Tauraco erythrolophus*
  Lower left: Carmine bee-eater, *Merops nubicus*
  Upper right: Racquet-tailed roller, *Coracias spatulata*
  Lower right: Rose-crowned fruit dove, *Ptilinopus regina*

Published simultaneously in Canada and the United States by

HANCOCK HOUSE PUBLISHERS LTD.
19313 Zero Avenue, Surrey, B.C. V4P 1M7
(604) 538-1114   Fax (604) 538-2262

HANCOCK HOUSE PUBLISHERS
1431 Harrison Avenue, Blaine, WA 98230-5005
(604) 538-1114   Fax (604) 538-2262

Contents

Acknowledgments 9
Introduction 10
1 Acclimating and Establishing 11
    Birds Imported from the Wild 11
    Captive-bred and Established Birds 13
    Transferring Outdoors 14
2 Purchasing a Softbill 16
    Questions to Ask on the Phone 16
    Personal Visit 16
    Visual Inspection 17
    Close Inspection in the Hand 18
3 Housing 21
    Flight Cages 21
    The Outdoor Aviary 23
    The House 23
    The Outside Flight 26
    Indoor Aviaries 28
    Tubular Framed Aviaries 30
4 Plants 31
    Indoor Aviaries 31
    Outdoor Aviaries 32
    Hanging Baskets 33
    Plants Considered Safe 34
    Potentially Toxic Plants 34

5	Catching and Handling	36
	Catching from Aviaries	36
	Catching from Cages	37
	Handling	37
6	Diets and Feeding Techniques	39
	Softbill Food	40
	Live Foods	43
	Softbill Diets	50
7	Nutrition	58
	Proteins, Fats and Carbohydrates	58
	Drinking and Bathing Water	61
	Vitamins and Minerals	62
	Vitamins	62
	Minerals	68
	Mineral Inhibitors	72
8	Breeding	73
	Sexing	73
	Breeding Environment	75
	Breeding Stimuli	76
	Nesting Receptacles	78
	Nesting Materials	80
	Rearing	81
	Breeding Problems	83
9	Rings, Records and Studbooks	85
	Leg Bands	85
	Records	86
	Studbooks	87
10	Incubation and Hand Rearing	89
	Incubation	89
	The Incubator	90
	The Incubation Process	93
	Hand Rearing	97

Hygiene	97
Immediately after Hatching	98
Food	99
Feeding	100
Fruit Pigeons and Doves	103
Problems during Hand Feeding	103
References	105

11 Ailments . . . 107

Treatment	107
Hygiene	108
Disinfectants	110
Droppings and Their Diagnostic Value	110
Botulism	112
Aspergillosis	112
Candidiasis (*Candida albicans*)	113
Salmonella	114
Antibiotics as a Prophylactic	115
Escherichia coli	115
Coccidiosis	116
Pseudotuberculosis (Yersiniosis)	117
Worms	117
Mites and Lice	118
Bumblefoot	119
Gangrene	120
Iron-Storage Disease	120
Rickets	121
Night Frights	122
Probiotics—A Prophylactic	122
Common Ailments	124
Acknowledgments	124
References	124
Further Reading	124
Table of Common Ailments	125

12 Species Accounts 127
    Tanagers 177
    Euphonias and Chlorophonias 180
    Honeycreepers 183
    Pekin Robin and Silver-eared Mesia 185
    Laughing Thrushes 188
    Fairy Bluebirds 190
    Chloropsis 193
    White Eyes (Zosterops) 196
    Sunbirds and Spiderhunters 199
    Shama and Dhyal Thrushes 203
    Pittas 206
    Old World Flycatchers 209
    Broadbills 212
    Bulbuls 215
    Starlings, Mynahs and Oxpeckers 217
    Crows, Magpies and Jays 222
    Oropendolas 225
    Bee Eaters 228
    Rollers 232
    Hornbills 234
    Kingfishers and Kookaburras 238
    Toucans, Toucanets and Aracaris 241
    Barbets 245
    Hummingbirds 248
    Rails 252
    Shorebirds 255
    Touracos 260
    Fruit Pigeons and Doves 264
Diet Index 268
Index: Common and Scientific Names 272

Acknowledgments

I would like to thank my father, Colin Vince, for reading and adding a great deal to the text of this book, and for his tremendous encouragement throughout the project. Thank you especially to my wife, Renata, for reading the text and helping me with Americanisms, and for putting up with the endless evenings I spent at the computer or holding slides up to the light.

Very special thanks goes to Dr. Matt Dahlquist, DVM for giving so much of his time to correct and improve both the nutrition and ailments chapters. They turned out very well and I couldn't have done them on my own—thank you.

Thank you to Dave Rimlinger, Curator of Birds at the San Diego Zoo, for helping me identify the picture of the rufous laughing thrush. And thank you to Raul and Elsa Cruz for helping with all my computer questions.

Thank you also to all of my friends at Sedgwick County Zoo, Wichita, Kansas, and Riverbanks Zoo and Garden, Columbia, South Carolina. I have learned much at both institutions and continue to greatly enjoy working as the Assistant Curator of Birds at Riverbanks.

The art department at Riverbanks Zoo and Garden has been very kind in letting me reproduce some of their photographs in this book. For that I am most grateful. And I particularly want to thank Bob Seibels, Curator of Birds at the Riverbanks Zoo and Garden, for giving me free access to his personal library of slides. They add considerable quality to the book.

Introduction

What is a softbill?

"Softbill" is a general term used by aviculturists to describe a wide range of small, flying birds. They do not actually have soft beaks, but merely live on soft foods like fruit, nectar or insects; as opposed to "hardbills," such as parrots and finches, that live mainly on seeds and nuts. Many softbills eat more than 1 food type, and some, such as magpies and jays, will include tiny birds and amphibians in their diet. In spite of their often varied tastes, softbills can be divided into 4 distinct dietary categories:

    omnivore—most foods are eaten;
    insectivore—mainly insects are eaten;
    frugivore—mainly fruits are eaten;
    nectivore—mainly nectar is eaten.

To every rule there are exceptions, and the definition of a softbill is no different. Lories and lorikeets are birds that live on nectar and fruits but are actually classified as parrots. And some of the falconets with their purely insectivorous lifestyles could be called softbills, but instead are birds of prey.

The definition of a softbill is a somewhat subjective one, and it depends on avicultural instinct as much as any hard and fast rules; but generally: softbills are small, flying birds that do not live on seed, but at least one of the following: fruit, insects, nectar or meat.

1

Acclimating and Establishing

Birds Imported from the Wild

Acclimating and establishing are 2 vital processes that must go hand in hand to bring a bird safely from the wild into captivity, and these processes should largely be achieved during quarantine. While the need for acclimation is well known, the purpose and value of establishing a softbill is often overlooked. This process, which involves readjusting the bird to captive conditions, must be done correctly or losses can be high.

Before reaching the importer, a softbill is likely to have suffered a considerable ordeal from its capture and throughout the long transportation process. Although food and water do accompany birds on international flights, the noise, movement, temperature changes and constant commotion dissuade all but the briefest of feedings. Softbills therefore often arrive thin, stressed and sick.

From day 1

For the first week of quarantine a softbill is best kept at about 85°F (29.4°C). This should approximate to the temperature in the wild and will also prevent an excessive loss of body heat, acting almost like a hospital cage.

Encouraging the birds to feed during the first few hours is crucial and usually the key to success—with their often small bodies and high metabolisms, softbills can otherwise quickly succumb. It is imperative that the food offered to the birds be as enticing as possible. Foods frequently suitable for established softbills can be useless for newly imported ones, since pellets and the like will appear inedible to birds that only days before may have been in the wild. Fruit pieces must be clearly visible and not smothered with artificial foods. Plenty of live food should be given to insectivores for the first month to replace lost body weight; and for nectivores, the outlets of nectar tubes and bottles should be clearly marked with a ring of red paint or a red plastic flower. Room lights should be left on for the first night and dull night lights should be employed thereafter.

From day 7

After about a week, the birds should be settled and more receptive to artificial foods. Gradually the fruit content of the omnivore and frugivore diets can be reduced and replaced with the more nutritious proprietary foods, until the correct maintenance diet is established. Insectivores too will begin to eat the proprietary food during quarantine. However to fully establish them, "meating-off" techniques may have to be used once the quarantine is complete. (See Diets on page 39.)

Throughout the quarantine process, the temperature should be gradually reduced until by the final week, the softbills are accustomed to about 65°F (18.3°C). The acclimating and establishing process is now largely complete. During appropriate weather the softbills can be transferred to outdoor aviaries.

Medicating

Inevitably some softbills die in quarantine and it is vital that an autopsy be performed immediately. The remainder of the birds can then be medicated on the assumption that they are also infected. Unfortunately, such laboratory work takes a few days and the delay is often costly, especially for small softbills such as bananaquits, hummingbirds, sunbirds, tits, warblers, wrens, white eyes and yuhinas. It is therefore beneficial to assume the birds are suffering from some kind of pathogen from the outset, and employ a blanket probiotic treatment from day one. (See Probiotics on page 123 and Salmonella on page 114.)

Housing

Stress can severely hinder the establishing process and will greatly exacerbate an illness. However, stress can be substantially minimized by housing birds according to their individual personalities.

In aviaries many species can be housed together for the duration of the quarantine, but beware of overcrowding—even sociable birds such as Pekin robins, *Leiothrix lutea*, will pluck each other's napes bare if too closely confined.

Certain softbills, such as most insectivores, thrushes, sunbirds and hummingbirds, are pugnacious by nature and need to be housed individually. Ideally, the birds should be kept in small, solid, wire-fronted cages. Even if such birds lived as pairs with their previous owner, unless they can be quarantined in aviaries or very large cages, house them separately to be on the safe side. Stress may be lowered if they cannot see each other and generally a visual barrier between enclosures is helpful for all birds in quarantine.

Captive-bred and Established Birds

Even if a bird is captive bred and has already been established elsewhere, when it arrives at your facility it should be treated as a newly imported specimen. On arrival it will need to be quarantined, and the new owner should take account of its stressed, tired and frightened condition.

Quarantine is essential to help protect your collection and should last a minimum of 1 month, longer if there are any problems. This is especially important for softbills, because after quarantine they are often kept in planted aviaries with soil floors. In this kind of environment it can be very difficult to completely remove disease-causing microorganisms once they have been introduced—replacing the soil and vegetation is usually the only option.

During quarantine, cages or aviaries with solid sides and backs will provide a secluded environment, making the birds feel safer and more inclined to feed. Ideally, new birds should be housed singly or in small groups so that their food consumption can be accurately monitored. Health checks are also much easier with smaller groups, and your veterinarian may do a fecal examination to check for common problems such as worms and Coccidia.

A quarantine temperature of 65°–70°F is usually sufficient for softbills that are not newly imported. Night lights are beneficial until the new arrival has settled down and is feeding normally. Fruits must be clearly visible and plenty of insects should be provided until the standard maintenance diet is accepted. If the softbill takes a long time to settle down and is not feeding properly, introduce a bird of the same or similar species to the cage. The newly purchased bird should feel more relaxed and start feeding alongside the established one. Remember that the quarantine will have to start anew from the day the "teacher" bird is introduced.

Transferring Outdoors

Completing the acclimation process can take as long as a year and usually begins in the summer months when the weather is warmest and daylight hours are longest. It is then that the softbill can be transferred to the outdoor aviary; experiencing no appreciable change in temperature, the move is comfortable and safe. The softbill is still fairly delicate at this stage and transferring outdoors during cold weather is likely to fail.

Initially the softbill is confined to the house part of the aviary for several days. It will then associate the house with warmth, security and, most important of all, food and water. But once given access to the flight, it will probably not have enough sense to roost in the house and may be in danger. It is therefore necessary to chase the bird into the house each evening and lock it in, repeating the process over several consecutive evenings. After about a week of this routine, the bird usually learns to roost in the house and no longer needs to be chased in.

When introducing a bird to an established group, a small release ("howdie") cage may be used. The bird should be caged for several days and can be positioned in the house or flight. If there is no aggression shown by any of the other birds, the new one can be released, with plenty of food and water in full view until the bird settles in. Adding new branches or plants can help disrupt established territories and assuage future aggression from existing birds.

For birds in outdoor aviaries, a night light is particularly valuable—a dull bulb of about 10 watts, or old Christmas tree lights, can be used to illuminate the shelter. This will allow birds to continue feeding through the night and survive low or even freezing temperatures. Softbills panicked by storms, vermin or other commotions can find a perch more easily without colliding into walls and injuring themselves.

Winter—delicate species

Winter can bring freezing temperatures to many regions of the world and in these conditions delicate softbills need a heated house. Here they will spend much of the winter, being given access to the flight on only unseasonably warm days. If a heated shelter is not available, the less-hardy species will need to be removed to winter quarters such as a heated bird room.

Delicate or semidelicate species include barbets, broadbills, chats, euphonias, flycatchers, fruit pigeons, honeycreepers, hummingbirds, *Chloropsis*, manakins, motmots, pittas, redstarts, spiderhunters, sunbirds, most tanagers, tits, white eyes, woodpeckers and yuhinas.

Winter—hardy species

There are a number of softbills that can live without heat. In all but the worst of weather, they can be given regular access to their outdoor flight during the day and shut into a frost-free house at night. Generally, provided they are healthy and well fed, such birds can tolerate near-freezing temperatures.

Hardy species include babblers, drongos, large honeyeaters, large hornbills, jays, kiskadees, magpies, Pekin robin, large shrikes, large sibias, silver-eared mesia, starlings, thrushes, and blue-gray and mountain tanagers.

Diet

Softbills being wintered-out in the absence of heat must have extra carbohydrates in their diet. Soaked sultanas, mashed boiled potatoes and grated cheese will all help fuel the body through almost-freezing temperatures, but by spring these foods should be removed from the diet to prevent obesity. For the more delicate species overwintered in heated accommodation, dietary modifications are not necessary provided temperatures exceed about 55°F (13°C).

One year later, the acclimation process is complete. Having experienced the full range of temperatures which can be safely tolerated, the softbills are now as acclimated as they will ever be.

2

Purchasing a Softbill

Questions to Ask on the Phone

The seller is unlikely to volunteer information that might jeopardize the sale, so the following points should be covered to get a true picture of the bird:

1. Captive bred or wild caught?
2. Sex; if dimorphic, is it old enough to be sexed visually? If monomorphic, has surgical or laboratory sexing been carried out and by whom? Ask to see the veterinary report.
3. Age; is it post or prereproductive?
4. General condition; injuries, medical history, veterinary treatment. Is the bird now fully recovered?
5. Is it aggressive to cage mates; has it caused death or injury?
6. Why is it for sale; genuine reason?
7. Has it bred and successfully raised young in the last two years?
8. Vices; does it eat its own eggs or pluck its young? These vices can be practically impossible to cure. (See Breeding Problems.)
9. Why is a good breeding bird for sale?

Personal Visit

It is always advisable to see a bird before purchasing it. A personal visit allows a thorough examination of the softbill, as well as an opportunity to see its diet and environment. A healthy bird is usually easy to recognize: it stands erect, and is sleek, bright eyed and lively. An unhealthy one may not be so easy to identify, but some of the more obvious illnesses can be ruled out following a careful inspection.

Visual Inspection

Plumage

Newly imported softbills will often look scruffy, having been repeatedly handled and perhaps overcrowded. The roughness of their feathers should not give undue cause for concern, however; an otherwise healthy bird will soon molt into beauty. Good nutrition and fresh bathing water are especially important at this time, and softbills with an incomplete plumage should be kept warmer than normal until fully feathered.

Breathing

Labored breathing, often characterized by tail bobbing, may indicate a respiratory infection; a veterinary examination will almost certainly be needed. Open-mouthed breathing should also be treated with suspicion since Aspergillosis or a *Candida* infection could be to blame. The whitish fungus of candidiasis may be seen inside the mouth and prompt treatment is usually successful. Nectivores are said to be particularly at risk—as high levels of sugar in their diet seem to encourage the fungus—although most softbills are vulnerable. Aspergillosis is a very serious disease; it is difficult to cure and often only confirmed by an autopsy. (See Ailments—Aspergillosis.)

Nostrils

Blocked nostrils can also cause breathing problems. Check that there is no discharge and that the nostrils are clear and of equal size to rule out the possibility of a localized infection. Nasal discharge may be caused by something innocuous like a great change in the environmental temperature. However, it is likely to be more complex and can be caused by many things such as a viral or bacterial infection, and even aspergillosis. A simple inspection will not give the answer and laboratory work will need to be done by your veterinarian. Even then, if an infection has extended into the sinuses, treatment can be very difficult and turn into a long-term project. Therefore, such birds make an uncertain purchase and should probably be avoided.

Some softbills are particularly messy feeders and plugs of dried food may accumulate in the nostrils. These blockages can be eased away with something like a toothpick. Lumps of food may also stick to the face and can be carefully removed after presoaking them in warm water.

Eyes

Conjunctivitis (pinkeye) is not uncommon in newly imported birds; the tissue surrounding the eye becomes a deep red and may be accompanied by a discharge. If only one eye is affected, an injury from a piece of dirt may be responsible. But if both eyes are involved, airborne dust or an infection could be the cause. Such infections often appear far worse than they actually are, and an ophthalmic ointment or drops prescribed by a veterinarian should effect a cure. My preference is for medication in the form of ointment, since drops are more easily washed out of the eye.

Potentially more serious, but less common, is a corneal abrasion. The damage to the cornea will often make the bird squint and can be caused by problems such as infection or trauma; or the injury may be self inflicted if the bird excessively rubs the eye. Treatment is normally with an antibiotic medication which is applied several times a day.

If both eyes are partly closed the softbill may simply be drowsy. A healthy bird will normally relax on one leg; sleeping or resting on both legs is likely to indicate poor health. With red-eyed birds examine their eyes very carefully since they are more prone to blindness and cataracts than dark-eyed species.

Close Inspection in the Hand

Cosmetics

Examining the bird of your choice in the hand will allow a more meaningful inspection and will also highlight any cosmetic defects that may affect a career on the show bench. Missing or malformed claws, wings that are of unequal length or hung unevenly, a chipped or deformed bill and any other imperfections will all affect any judging, although these inadequacies will almost certainly have no bearing on the bird's breeding potential.

Body condition

A softbill's body condition can be roughly gauged by feeling the muscle tone on either side of its keel (breastbone). Although good muscle tone does not guarantee good health, its absence may well indicate an illness, especially in established birds. Newly imported softbills, however, are often thin but soon return to full weight if otherwise healthy.

External parasites

Mites and lice are external parasites and may secrete themselves in the plumage. They are found particularly around the vent and under the wings, and can cause tremendous irritation as affected birds often damage or pull out their feathers. Treatment is relatively easy with a suitable powder or spray. (See Ailments—mites and lice.)

Vent

Loose droppings are not a good sign and can have many causes such as a bacterial infection. Feathers around the vent may be stained by, or covered in, feces and the vent itself could be swollen. Immediate veterinary care is needed to replace lost fluids and nutrients. And a fresh stool specimen should be examined under the microscope to rule out internal parasites. Veterinary treatment will depend very much on the cause of the problem, with antibiotics often used to treat intestinal infections. Generally such birds are best avoided or purchased with great caution.

Feet

Finally, take a look at the bird's feet. In a dirty environment the tiniest abrasion can lead to bumblefoot; and although terrestrial species are most at risk, all softbills should be monitored. Bumblefoot appears as a soft swelling and should not be confused with gout which is similar in appearance but much harder to the touch. Bumblefoot can usually be cured, although at present no remedy exists for gout. (See also Ailments—bumblefoot.)

A more common problem among newly imported birds is accumulations of dried food and droppings that encase the toes or foot.

These may cut off the blood supply, resulting in dry gangrene and the loss of a toe. The deposits can fairly easily be broken away by first soaking the foot in warm water. Great care must be taken to prevent the accidental removal of a claw or an entire toe. An antiseptic cream should then be applied to seal any cracks and protect against infection. Vetbond (which is actually sterile superglue) is an excellent sealer of wounds that are likely to be reopened by regular use.

Arriving home

The change of diet and housing can be a traumatic time in a bird's life, and the transition from one owner to another must be done carefully. Most importantly, the bird should be quarantined before it is added to your collection. (See Acclimating and Establishing.)

3

Housing

Flight Cages

These cages represent the traditional way of housing softbills and are still popular as permanent housing for pets such as mynah birds. Large flight cages, as well as some indoor aviaries, often have bird rooms to provide temporary accommodation for sick or newly acquired birds, or breeding environments for very small species.

Building a flight cage

The flight cage is essentially a wooden box with a wire-mesh front, an entrance door and a sliding tray to remove droppings. The cage should be at least 3 ft. (90 cm) long x 1 ft. (30 cm) x 1 ft. (30 cm) to house a pair of white-eye-sized birds or a single softbill the size of a bulbul. For something as big as a mynah bird, the cage will need to be twice as large in every dimension to prevent obesity.

The wood used in construction of the cage should be nonabsorbent or well painted to protect it from wet droppings. Naturally messy feeding habits and fondness for bathing are typical of most softbills. Melamine-covered chipboard is ideal, being tough and easy to clean.

A flat, sliding tray at the bottom of the cage allows the droppings to be removed without disturbing the softbill. The tray is fitted with a front edge and handle so it can be pulled forward like a drawer. Aluminum is the best material, since wooden sheets quickly warp when wet.

The cage front can be homemade from a panel of wire mesh or a ready-made front, with a sliding door, can be purchased and easily fitted. Sliding doors tend to be better when keeping small, fast softbills since they can be opened without being hinged forward; this reduces escapes which are minimized further by locating doors close to the floor, below perch level.

Perches

Tree branches of between 0.5 in. (1.2 cm) and 1.5 in. (3.6 cm) diameter can be used for large softbills, while for the smaller species, thinner perches with more side shoots are best. Branches may be contaminated by wild birds' droppings, pollution or pesticides, and should be disinfected and thoroughly dried before use.

Perches should be fixed firmly, otherwise breeding can be affected. The selected branch can be sharpened to a point at one end and split with a knife at the other. The sharpened end is pressed into a small hole drilled into the back of the cage, while the split end is pressed into the wire-mesh front. This fixes the perch securely while allowing easy removal or replacement.

A perch should be positioned at each end of the flight cage, allowing enough room for the softbill to turn easily without damaging its tail. Do not fix the perches too low. The higher the perch, the more secure the bird will tend to feel. Additional perches may be added but do not clutter the cage: exercise is essential and the softbill will need to fly uninterrupted the full length of the flight cage to remain fit.

Most softbills have fairly soft feet, and fresh, clean perches are essential for good health. Perches can quickly become contaminated by feces and fruit pieces; minor cuts or abrasions caused by hard perching or an injury can soon lead to bumblefoot. Dowel perches are popular but not recommended because they are generally too hard and potentially abrasive. Equally, their constant diameter cannot exercise the foot muscles and toes as well as the varying surfaces of natural wood.

Floor covering

Two or 3 sheets of newspaper make the most practical floor covering for a softbill cage since they can be frequently and cheaply replaced—tape them together or weigh the sheets down with food bowls to prevent them from blowing away.

Sand and sawdust should be avoided as floor coverings. Sand

may be abrasive and harmful to the feet of terrestrial species, while the down draft of beating wings can cloud sawdust into the air and may cause eye or respiratory problems. Also, both materials can stick to food and be accidentally ingested.

The Outdoor Aviary

Generally, softbill aviaries are designed in much the same way as those for other birds. Particular attention is given to the house part, since in a temperate climate all softbills need winter protection with many requiring heat.

Site planning

When choosing a site for the aviary, take advantage of existing structures or vegetation: a tall garden wall, trees and hedges all help shield the aviary from severe weather. They also help it blend in attractively with its surroundings. Beware of very large trees, however, since their roots can undermine an aviary's foundation, and in a storm, falling branches can cause serious damage. It can also be particularly gloomy under such trees and this will tend to subdue the birds and reduce their feeding activity.

The shelter may need electricity for heaters, lights and power sources. The installation must be done by a qualified electrician and the overall cost will be reduced if the aviary can be located near an existing supply, such as your house. Consult local planning regulations and even if building permits are not required, discuss the proposed aviary with your neighbors to preserve good relations. Avoid building near a road. Thieves can gain easy access to the aviary; or the passing traffic might upset your birds, especially if they are trying to breed.

The House

Dimensions

The house must be large enough to accommodate all of the birds for lengthy periods, since during winter the less-hardy species will spend more time in the house than outside. The building should be easily sanitized and should also be bright, otherwise the birds will be reluctant to use it. The dimensions of the house depend on the number and species of softbills being kept, and the available budget. But as an example: a house of only 4 ft. (1.2 m) x 2 ft. (0.6 m) x 6 ft. (1.8 m) high can serve a flight of 10 ft. (3 m) x 4 ft. (1.2 m) x 7 ft. (2.1 m) high. This will accommodate a pair of starling-sized birds and should be sufficient for them to breed.

Foundation

A concrete foundation will be needed to support the structure and help deter vermin such as mice, rats, raccoons and foxes. If the house is to be made of wood, build up the base with brick to raise the framework off the ground. This will help prevent rotting and will also look more attractive.

Insulation

Insulation is vital in a softbills' shelter, giving protection from subzero winters as well as dangerously hot summers. The gap between the inner and outer walls can be filled with insulating material, or the gap alone may provide sufficient insulation. Take care not to leave any small holes through which mice and other vermin could gain entry. They have a great liking for wall cavities and, once in, are extremely difficult to eradicate.

Roof

A flat roof is relatively easy to make and should slope to the rear of the building, preferably toward a gutter. Thick plywood covered with shingles or tiles looks very attractive. To conserve heat, the loft should be filled with an insulating material.

Lighting

Artificial: nervous or breeding birds can be easily panicked by sudden movements seen through a window. For sensitive specimens, four solid walls and artificial lighting may be best. Full-spectrum Vitalites™ provide good quality lighting and produce the ultraviolet wavelengths necessary for vitamin D_3 synthesis (which the body needs for calcium absorption). To receive the full benefits of the artificial ultraviolet light, the birds must usually be within about 3 ft. (0.9 m) of the source. (See Nutrition—vitamin D_3.)

Natural: for relatively calm birds, a south-facing window can offer good lighting and, when screened, can be opened to provide valuable ventilation to help prevent diseases like aspergillosis. (See Ailments—aspergillosis.) An open window can also expose your birds to direct sunlight which the body needs for vitamin D_3 synthesis.

Screening the window also identifies it as solid which will prevent newly introduced birds from trying to fly through it. If screening is not used, the glass will need to be temporarily marked with tape or streaks of soap. After a few days the birds should be used to the window and the markings can be gradually removed.

Night lights: these are extremely important but often overlooked. A 10-watt light bulb or a string of old Christmas tree lights left on during the night will allow a bird to find a perch without injuring itself. Birds can also feed through the night which is especially important in low temperatures and during acclimation. (See Acclimating and Establishing; and Ailments—night frights.)

Safety porch

As you enter the aviary, fast softbills can easily escape, and even fairly tame birds quickly become disoriented, frightened and increasingly difficult to recapture. A safety porch, with its double-door system, is therefore highly recommended. Although a porch can be built onto the outdoor flight, the aviary will look much tidier if it is made a part of the house. An enlarged porch can also be used to store food and equipment or sectioned off to make a bird room. This is the ideal location for a food preparation area along with cages and small aviaries for additional breeding pairs, new arrivals and juveniles from last year's breeding season.

Heating

Many softbills need heat during the winter. This can be provided by tubular heaters which are cheap, safe, easy to install and available in a range of wattages. They can be positioned fairly near the floor to thoroughly heat the room. But if they are in the shelter, birds will tend to stand on them; therefore, a metal cover sloping sharply downwards from the wall may be needed to avoid burned feet.

Air quality

Good ventilation is important in any enclosed space where birds are kept. Warm, damp air that is allowed to become stagnant will promote the growth of fungal spores which under certain conditions may become pathogenic. (See Ailments—Aspergillosis.) Airborne spores and dust should be minimized by using an extractor fan or an air purification unit that is large enough to achieve a regular change of air.

One might also consider purchasing an ionizer when attempting to achieve good air quality. Ionizers are devices that remove dust and bacteria from the atmosphere by producing negative ions. Studies have shown that the ions actually destroy harmful bacteria, reducing the atmospheric bacterial count by up to 90 percent in one hour. In the United States, units are available which use ozone, as well as negative ions, to purify the air. A range of such machines is distributed by Pure 'n' Natural Systems, 52-B Cummings Park, Suite 311, Woburn, MA, 01801.

In the U.K., air filtration units that incorporate ionizers are available from Innovations Ltd., Euroway Business Park, Swindon, Wiltshire, SN5 8SN.

The Outside Flight

Foundation

The flight is usually constructed of timber, and like the house, will be longer lasting and more attractive if built on a low wall. The wall's concrete foundation will also help deter vermin from digging into the aviary and threatening the health of your collection. When building the foundation it is a good idea to bury gravel on either side of it to assist drainage and prevent large pools of rain water from accumulating in the flight.

Framework

The flight itself is essentially a number of prefabricated frames, fixed onto the wall and bolted to each other—this sectional method of construction is easy and allows the aviary to be dismantled if you move house. When the timber framework is first assembled, it can be very unstable without the wire mesh to strengthen it. Temporary supports are highly recommended, especially if the flight is very large or likely to be affected by strong winds.

Once the framework is in place the wire mesh can be fitted, but before this is done be sure that the interior of the flight is complete with plants, perches, pools, etc. Such items can be difficult to introduce when the only point of entry is the safety porch.

Roof

Softbills and especially their nests can be greatly affected by a sudden downpour. Covering half of the roof with transparent plastic sheeting provides valuable protection. Rain can then fall through the other half of the roof to water the plant-life. But before fitting the roofing sheets, it is preferable to first cover the entire roof with wire mesh. This will prevent escapes if the sheeting is ripped off during a storm. As it gets older, plastic sheeting becomes brittle; material treated against ultraviolet light tends to last longer.

Perch heaters

Most birds become used to roosting in their house, but some inevitably do not. This can be a particular problem in the winter when freezing conditions may cause injuries such as frost-bitten toes.

Perch heaters are made of a flexible tape, originally used as a method of warming pipes for the chemical industry. The tape contains a thermostatically controlled heating element, which is simple, cheap and safe, with the recommended power consumption of only 15 watts per foot. When the tape is clipped to the underside of a perch, the heat rises thereby keeping toes warm and protected.

Not every perch in the flight needs to be heated—just the higher ones, since they are mainly used for roosting.

Floor covering

In a small aviary, paving stones or concrete make an easily sanitized floor covering that can be decorated with plants in troughs and pots. Paving stones can also be used to form a pathway if frequent access to a flight is required.

Grass can greatly enhance an aviary's appearance and is obviously excellent for terrestrial softbills such as pittas and rails. Planting turf instead of seed can save a lot of time, and provided they are well watered for the first few weeks, soon become established. In the larger aviary, plants can be set in the ground, with much more natural results and often much faster growth.

A planted aviary certainly looks beautiful and is the best environment for your birds. A poorly designed aviary can be hard to keep clean. Accumulations of droppings on grass are impossible to remove without leaving a bare patch; so strategically position rocks or stones under favorite perches to make cleaning easier. Avoiding overcrowding is the very best way of keeping an aviary clean. With only a few birds in a relatively large area, daily cleaning will often not be necessary, except around food dishes. This means less work for the keeper, and more importantly, the reduced level of disturbance will promote breeding.

Indoor Aviaries

One of the main advantages of being indoors is protection from bad weather; a shelter is therefore not needed, and the aviary's general construction can be simpler and less substantial. Breeding programs can also be greatly assisted by the ability to manipulate photoperiods, rain cycles and temperature. (See also Breeding Stimuli.)

Mice, snakes, rats, raccoons, owls and foxes can all terrorize an outdoor aviary, and although vermin are ever-present, they are far easier to control within a building. Poisoning and trapping are usually effective preventative measures. Ultrasonic devices can be used to deter rodents. These devices produce a high-pitched sound that does not harm the birds, but affects the rodents' nervous system and produces considerable discomfort.

Greenhouses and conservatories

We have all seen the large tropical houses found in many modern zoos and wish to recreate in miniature our own jungle by converting an existing greenhouse or conservatory. The warm, humid environment easily created under glass is ideal for a variety of softbills, as well as the insects that many of them feed on. The tropical plants also provide excellent nest sites and nest-building materials.

Unfortunately such an aviary is often impractical as running costs can be prohibitive—key problems being those of heating and cooling. In the summer, keeping temperatures below an acceptable level of about 29°C (85°F) may be a problem; and heating a glass aviary during the winter can be equally difficult and expensive.

If effective heating and cooling can be achieved, the greenhouse will need additional work to make it safe for birds. The walls of a glass house can be dangerous since some birds will fly into them and are likely to be stunned or killed. To help prevent this, trees, bushes and climbing plants can be positioned in front of the glass. This will also help screen the building from harsh sunlight and help insulate it from the cold.

Large tropical houses

Introducing a new bird: adding a new bird to an existing collection should always be done carefully, but very special care must be taken when releasing a bird into an extremely large and well-planted enclosure. The softbill will need to familiarize itself with its new companions, and vice versa, but more importantly will have to quickly learn the geography of the facility and be made aware of its feeding opportunities.

A fairly large release cage should be positioned so that it is in full view of the other birds but located away from people. An aviary that is about 12 ft. (3.6 m) long will allow the bird to reach the necessary level of pre-release fitness. This is important, because once the softbill is released it will largely have to fend for itself, and will need a degree of fitness that may have been eroded by quarantine or life in a small cage.

The softbill will remain in the release cage for one or two weeks so that it can settle into its new environment and see other birds feeding from nearby dishes. When it is released, the new bird will then be able to find food locally, in an area that is already familiar. The release itself must be as stress-free as possible—simply open the door and walk away, do not chase the bird out.

Pools and drinking water: large enclosures will tend to have fairly deep, fast-flowing waters, presenting very real dangers to the birds inevitably drawn to them. Newly introduced birds are at particular risk since their ability to escape from the water may be impaired by a general lack of fitness.

Water dishes should be provided with the food, so that birds can drink and bathe in safety. This will also benefit very small species, like wrens, that cannot safely bathe in water more than a few centimeters deep, even when fully fit. (See Nutrition—drinking and bathing water.)

Pools in the smaller aviary: pools and streams are likely to be shallower with weaker flowing water; but these can still be dangerous, particularly to young fledglings which have only rudimentary flying skills and can easily drown. Because of the dangers, and the need for frequent cleaning, some aviculturists avoid streams and pools altogether. However, the considerable beauty of flowing water arguably outweighs the problems which are actually quite small and easy to overcome.

Shallow streams will have to be cleaned at least every second day, since feces, food and algae very quickly contaminate them. In warm weather, evaporation can also be a problem, and water will need to be dribbled into the system almost constantly.

Fledglings and drowning: pools and streams can be temporarily emptied or covered to safeguard fledglings. Where this is not possible or practical, such as in a public exhibit, the chicks may have to be hand reared. Alternately, the youngsters can be placed in a large cage at the time of fledging, and the parents will continue to feed them through the wire mesh.

Tubular Framed Aviaries

Aluminum 1 in. x 1 in. square tubing can be used to build the frames of aviaries and cages. The wire mesh is then fixed to the frame with self-tapping, sheet-metal screws. Kits are available for cages and aviaries, but building the accommodation yourself from scratch is much cheaper. The tubing is fairly easy to cut and even easier to assemble using a variety of plastic corner and T-pieces. California Cageworks Corporation, 3314 Burton Avenue, Burbank, CA, 91504, is just one of the many suppliers of the square, metal tubing and plastic connecting pieces, as well as various clips and door latches.

4

Plants

Plants are of tremendous value in the softbill aviary, giving protection from the weather and encouraging breeding. Trees and bushes offer excellent nesting sites, while climbers help to bring seclusion—all of the plant-life provides potentially valuable nesting materials. Dense foliage acts as a windbreak, helps to create shade and deflects rain from birds not sensible enough to use their shelter. Fruiting varieties can add to your birds' diet, and attract insects to the aviary. Not least of all, plants just look wonderful, and create a natural environment which tends to make the softbills feel relaxed and generally more healthy.

Indoor Aviaries

To create a secluded environment, 1 or 2 tall, potted trees can be positioned near the front of the aviary, forming a natural curtain between the birds and anything that may disturb them. The following are plant species suitable for a softbill aviary; most are fast growing, bushy and abundant in potential nesting sites.

Ficus benjamina **(weeping fig)**

The small berries of this species are popular with most softbills, especially tanagers that eat *Ficus* berries in the wild. Most *Ficus* species grow into substantial trees, and make good aviary plants, often being bushy and attractive. They prefer moderately damp soil and good, but indirect, sunlight. These are tropical plants that do best in a humid atmosphere and regular misting will keep them healthy.

Radermachera sinica **(emerald tree)**
The emerald tree is attractive and bushy, and easily grows to 6 ft. (1.8 m) in a roomy pot. An ideal aviary plant that can be cared for like a *Ficus*.

Fatshedera lizei **(tree ivy)**
The tree ivy is a vigorous plant and ideal for quickly foliating an aviary. It grows as high as 6 ft. (1.8 m) and will thrive in semi-shade, preferring warm, moist conditions.

Hibiscus rosa-sinensis **(Chinese hibiscus)**
In the wild this plant can grow up to 10 ft. (3 m) tall, and the pure species produces short-lived, red blooms. It is dense and bushy, and a very effective aviary plant which can tolerate full sun, but must be given plenty of water.

Spathiphyllum clevelandii **(peace lily)**
The peace lily grows tall and bushy enough to create the ideal visual barrier, with its attractive cream flowers appearing throughout the year. It is easy to maintain and needs slightly damp soil, thriving equally in bright or semi-shaded locations.

Outdoor Aviaries

The selection of plants for the outdoor aviary will naturally be influenced by climatic factors and so a visit to your local plant nursery will be worthwhile. The choice is huge, so the following are just a few useful varieties; they are also winter hardy, being resistant to snow and ice.

Hedges often attract nesting activity from smaller softbills and play host to numerous insects. Hedges can be trimmed to any shape and size, and make a great contribution to the outdoor aviary. American arbor vitae, *Thuja occidentalis*; common boxwood, *Buxus sempervirens*; and common privet, *Ligustrum vulgare,* are all hardy, and ideal hedge species. But do not use privet in aviaries of leaf-eating softbills, such as many tanagers, because it can be toxic.

A splash of color can be introduced with the yellow blooms of *Berberis hortorum*, a shrub that often grows up to 5 ft. (1.5 m) tall. The evergreen color of ivy, *Hedera helix*, can be used to cover an unsightly wall or fence. But this is another plant that can be toxic, so use it as a visual barrier outside the aviary or with frugivorous species such as fruit doves and mousebirds.

And if cats are a problem, they may be deterred by planting a thorny bush, such as hawthorn, against the outside of the flight.

Conifers provide good ground cover, the larger bushes offering excellent nesting sites. There are many beautiful varieties of all shapes and sizes, and since conifers are evergreen they remain in color year-round. These tough plants also make good windbreaks and effectively seclude the aviary.

Bamboo can bring variety to an aviary and looks even more striking if planted in small groups. A number of bamboo species are available which make good nesting sites while also looking somewhat exotic.

Hanging Baskets

Whether indoors or outdoors, hanging baskets create instant and portable foliage, as well as adding excellent nesting sites to the aviary. Summer blooms can liven up an outdoor flight, and when winter approaches, the baskets can be brought inside.

Chlorophytum comosum **(spider plant)**

Spider plants grow in varying degrees of light and are simple to propagate. The plantlets that hang from its arching roots can be cut off and replanted—growth is fast and successful at any time of year, with the plant at its best in a warm, moist atmosphere. A mature spider plant makes a particularly good visual barrier, since the mass of plantlets hanging beneath it serve to double its coverage. Suspended near the aviary floor, a dense bunch of plantlets provides ground cover for terrestrial softbills such as pittas.

Pelargonium domesticum **(geranium)**

The many geranium hybrids come in a variety of blooms, from white to a deep violet, with foliage as attractive to the human eye as it is to the nest-building softbill. Geraniums need plenty of water without being saturated.

Cissus rhomboidia **(grape ivy)**

This is a most tolerant indoor plant and is at home on a trellis or in a basket. It prefers warmth and humidity, and is excellent for the indoor aviary.

Plants Considered Safe

Acacia	Donkey tail	Natal plum
African violet	Dracaena	Norfolk Island pine
Aloe plant	Dragon tree	Palms
Baby's tears	Ferns	Peperomia
Bamboo	Figs: creeping,	Petunia
Begonia	rubber, fiddle leaf	Pittosporum
Bougainvillea	laurel leaf,	Prayer plant
Chickweed	weeping.	Purple passion
Christmas cactus	Gardenia	Rubber tree
Cissus	Grape ivy	Schefflera
(Kangaroo vine)	Hens and chickens	Sensitive plant
Coffee tree	Jade plant	Spider plant
Coleus	Kalanchoe	Swedish ivy
Corn plant	Magnolia	Thistle
Crab apple	Marigolds	Wandering Jew
Dandelion	Monkey plant	White clover
Dogwood	Nasturtium	Zebra plant

Potentially Toxic Plants

Avocado	Firethorn	Oak
Azalea	Foxglove	Oleander
Baneberry	Heliotrope	Periwinkle
Bean plants	Holly	Philodendrons
Bird of paradise	Honeysuckle	Pigweed
Bleeding heart	Hydrangea	Poison ivy and oak
Boxwood	Ivy	Pokeweed
Bracken fern	Jasmine	Privet
Buckthorn	Jerusalem cherry	Purple sesbane
Bulb flowers	Jimsonweed	Rain tree
(amaryllis, iris,	Lantana	Red maple
daffodil, narcissus,	Larkspur	Rhubarb leaves
hyacinth)	Lily-of-the-valley	Rhododendrons

Burdock	Locusts	Sandbox tree
Buttercup	Lupine	Skunk cabbage
Coffee plants	May apple	Sorrel
Cowslip	Milkweed	Snowdrop
Crown vetch	Mistletoe	Spurges
Dieffenbachia	Mock orange	Sweet pea
Elderberry	Monkshood	Tobacco
Eucalyptus	Morning glory	Vetch
Euonymus	Mountain laurel	Wattle
Flame tree	Nettles	White cedar
Felt plant	Nightshade	Yews

5

Catching and Handling

Catching from Aviaries

The hand net is by far the most common and quick method of capture, and for starling-sized birds the rim of the net should be about 10 in. (24 cm) in diameter. It should also be well padded to help soften the blow if the bird is accidentally struck during a catching attempt. Even a padded rim can inflict damage, and so the capture must be done as carefully as possible.

Your very presence in the aviary may cause alarm, so speed is of the essence. Try to make the catch as easy as possible by removing perches and plants. If the aviary has a separate shelter, isolate the softbill by locking the unwanted birds into the house or flight.

It may be possible to slowly approach the softbill and net it on the wire mesh. But it is more likely the bird will fly past your shoulder to the other end of the aviary, remaining as high and distant as it can. This will allow the softbill's preferred flight-path to be seen and its movements more easily predicted.

Hold the net in one hand but do not raise it. With the other arm outstretched, walk toward the softbill and if the previous flight-path is repeated, quickly raise the net to catch the bird in midflight. Some precision is needed for an in-flight catch; and it may be easier to follow the softbill through the air, capturing it immediately after it lands on the wire mesh and before it has time to orientate itself.

As the bird begins to tire it will lose altitude and perhaps land on the floor. Although capture now becomes fairly easy, the stressed and panting softbill will be in no condition to undergo anything that could add to the stress, such as a lengthy veterinary examination. For some species a prolonged catch can be dangerous or even fatal, especially if they are ill.

The curtain net is a very fast method of capture that works well in a small aviary. The "net" is a large piece of material or netting that is as high and wide as the aviary itself. Once you are inside the aviary, hold the net up to the roof so that it hangs down to the floor and effectively partitions the flight. Walk the net toward the softbill and push it up against the end of the aviary to effect an easy capture. This is particularly useful for catching small, fast species, provided the aviary is first cleared of obstacles such as plants and perches.

The trap cage can be used in well-planted aviaries where a hand net or curtain net is unsuitable. The trap can be a small aviary or cage, operated automatically or simply by pulling a piece of string. In a mixed collection, a nonautomatic mechanism is best to avoid catching birds at random.

To overcome the birds' natural wariness, leave the trap open, unattended and with fresh food in it for a few days—they will soon learn to use the trap and can easily be caught. If the required bird does not enter the cage alone, spring the trap anyway, since another opportunity may be a long time in coming.

Catching from Cages

This is best done with the bare hand or a small aquarist's net. The process is similar to catching birds from the aviary: remove perches to allow the hand or net unobstructed movement and watch for the bird's preferred flight path. When your hand enters the cage, the softbill will usually fly to the cage front where the net or cupped hand can be ready.

Handling

The softbill will need to be removed carefully from the net and if necessary its claws unhooked one-by-one from the material. Be aware that some species have astonishingly strong feet, while others have bills that are capable of drawing blood.

Hold the softbill firmly and always be prepared for a sudden, wriggling motion that in unseasoned hands usually leads to an escape.

Stress: catching and holding most softbills will induce some fear and stress, but the period of restraint is usually brief, causing no harm at all. However, if you are worried about the amount of stress your bird may suffer while in the hand, perhaps during long procedures such as beak trimming, a herbal remedy can be used. Valerian is a common herbal sedative available from most health food stores and should be added to the bird's water for a few days before the procedure; valerian herbal tea is just as good.

Stress-molt: some feathers may become ruffled or fall out after handling, particularly if your hands are damp. In certain birds, however, a stress-molt can be induced and a surprising amount of feathers may be lost. This is a defense mechanism that would leave a predator chewing on a mouthful of feathers rather than the bird; and for softbills such as touracos, fruit doves and fruit pigeons, very careful handling is necessary. If the softbill is already confined in a box or small cage, catching it in complete darkness will help prevent a stress-molt. Do not extend this practice to catching birds from the aviary, since darkness and the use of a flashlight is bound to cause injury.

6

Diets and Feeding Techniques

The modern pelletized foods have given us nutritionally excellent diets that are easy and quick to prepare. And with improved nutrition has come the regular breeding of many softbills previously considered difficult to breed. But for all the technology, an understanding of your birds' feeding habits is still essential.

Ready-made foods can only form the foundation of a softbill diet, since pellets alone do not necessarily provide the correct nutrition for softbills; or the softbill pellet will not be eaten in its original form and will have to be ground up or moistened to be made palatable. So, as well as the proprietary foods, the vast majority of softbills need additional foods such as fruits, vegetables, insects, mice and small fish. The key is to feed each item in moderation and achieve a balanced intake.

It is a good idea to vary some of the ingredients in a diet within the natural feeding habits of the softbill—fruits can be varied according to what is cheap and in season. The variety will provide psychological enrichment, but more importantly, will help ensure proper nutrition.

A good diet should enable a bird to live for a long time, molt uneventfully and in good color, vocalize regularly and reach breeding condition at the normal time.

A personal anecdote

Recently I went to South America to collect a number of ramphastids (toucans) and psittacines (parrots) which were to become the founder members of a captive-breeding program. Many had already been assembled before my arrival; and although their condition looked good, the ramphastids were strangely motionless, and looked like stuffed exhibits in a museum. For three weeks they had been fed only bananas with drinking water offered in an old tin can.

From the local market I bought a water melon, star fruits, mangoes, papayas, hamburger (minced beef) and bread. The bread was soaked in a homemade nectar—sugar, powdered milk, milk shake and hot, bottled water—and then squeezed until fairly dry. This soaked bread made up 40 percent of the ramphastid diet, 50 percent was chopped fruits, and 10 percent was hamburger.

All of the birds thrived from that point on, with the aracaris eagerly hopping onto the food dish as soon as it touched the cage floor. And to help their general condition, larger water dishes were provided to allow bathing, as well as easier drinking.

Softbill Food

Proprietary softbill pellets

Pelletized foods provide an excellent, nutritious foundation for your softbill's diet. Generally, a small pellet (about the size of canary seed) is ideal, since it sticks to fruits and is automatically ingested.

One of the best pelletized diets for softbills and finches is called Tropical Bits, manufactured by Marion Zoological, P.O. Box 875, Wayzata, MN, 55391. These particular pellets are so tiny they can even be fed to the smallest insectivores, such as tits and wrens, without having to be powdered in a food processor. They also contain red and yellow-colored food that bring out the best in a bird's plumage. However, none of the pelletized diets is perfect, and in my opinion Tropical Bits have a tendency to cause thin-shelled eggs when the birds do not have access to direct sunlight. This is not a serious problem and vitamin D_3 supplementation or access to ultraviolet lighting appears to provide the solution.

Once acclimated, softbills of starling size and upwards, will comfortably swallow, round 7-mm diameter pellets. But my personal preference is to avoid such large foods, since I recently saw a Sulawesi king starling, *Basilornis celebensis*, feed a dry, 7 mm pellet to a nine-day-old chick. The chick was not harmed, although it could easily have been, even if I had soaked the pellets beforehand.

In Europe, good softbill foods such as Sluis and Prosecto can be bought from most pet stores. And in the recipes for softbill diets described in this chapter, such foods can be used instead of the "powdered/proprietary softbill pellet."

Fruits

Almost everything from tomatoes and bananas to star fruits and pears can be used, provided they are of good quality, fresh and properly ripened. Apples are available year round and are usually cheap, but use only dessert apples since cooking apples can be too acidic. Bananas are also quite cheap and a good food for softbills. Sometimes bananas are described as toxic; in large quantities, underripe and overripe bananas can cause digestive disturbances or even death in very small birds. But over the last 20 years, I have always found them to be perfectly safe when they constitute only 10 to 15 percent (by volume) of a balanced diet. Oranges can also cause digestive disturbances, but, like bananas, in moderation are a safe and valuable food.

Tomatoes are often popular and can be especially useful for tempting newly purchased birds to feed—the red color seems to attract them. Pears, mangoes, papayas, melons, pomegranates, cherries, peaches and any of the edible berries are all ideal for the softbill diet. Avocados are also favored by some aviculturists; but be aware of their dangerously high levels of lipids and vitamin E. The leaves and stem of the avocado plant are also potentially toxic. (See warning under vitamin E page 67.)

Dried fruits

Raisins, prunes, dried apricots and dried figs should be soaked for two hours in water and thoroughly rinsed under running water before feeding. Dried fruits are usually enjoyed by most birds but are high in calories and can be very fattening. Large amounts of dried fruits can also contribute to iron-storage disease and should not exceed 5 percent (by volume) of the entire diet. (See Ailments—iron-storage disease.) In fact, their value is greatest for birds wintered outdoors as described in transferring outdoors on page 14.

Vegetables

Boiled maize, peas, cucumber, cooked root vegetables, lettuce and even dandelion and chickweed are all very beneficial foods. Spinach can also be included; but it is high in oxalic acid and should be used carefully. (See Nutrition—mineral inhibitors.)

Hard-boiled eggs

This is an excellent food for all softbills since it contains all of the nutrients needed to form a chick. The egg should be mashed or very finely chopped, especially for insectivores which usually feed on the albumen quite eagerly; it presumably resembles foods such as wax moth larvae (waxworms) and ant pupae which are relished by the vast majority of softbills.

The structural compound of egg shells is calcium carbonate. Some aviculturists grind up the shells and include them in the diet as a calcium supplement. A balanced diet of softbill pellets, fruits, vegetables and insects is unlikely to need supplementation. But if it does, my preference is to use a manufactured vitamin or mineral supplement such as those made by Nekton™.

Color foods

Many birds can lose the vibrancy of their red, yellow or orange plumage after successive molts in captivity; troupials, minivets, trogons and certain bee eaters are just some of the softbills that can be affected. Natural pigment occurs in foods that are high in carotenes (orange to red-colored hydrocarbons found in many plants). The yellow carotenoid pigment (xanthophyll) is found in foods such as egg yolk and dark green vegetables, while red pigment (beta carotene) can be found in carrots, tomatoes, paprika, red peppers, sweet potatoes and red berries.

Nowadays, more potent, synthetic products are commercially available, like canthaxanthin, which is a red color food. Nekton™ U.S.A., Inc., Clearwater, Florida, distributes red and yellow color food which should also be available in the U.K.; and similar products are sold by John E. Haith, Cleethorpes, South Humberside, U.K.

Color feeding should start several weeks before the molt; and it should continue through the molt and for a short time afterward. As the new feathers grow, they receive the coloring agent in the blood supply and achieve their proper color. There are certain proprietary softbill and finch pellets such as Tropical Bits that already contain color food, and with these diets color feeding is not necessary. (See Proprietary Softbill Pellets.)

Freezing food

Grapes, pitted plums, peaches and most berries can be frozen. Spread them out on a tray so that none of the fruits touch each other, and put the tray in the freezer. Once they are frozen, the fruits can be transferred to a plastic container; they can then be defrosted individually instead of in one great lump. Most vegetables can also be frozen although they usually have to be blanched in boiling water first. (See Nutrition—drinking and bathing water.)

Live Foods

Mealworms, *Tenebrio molitor*

This is the larval form of the meal beetle and not actually a worm. It is a popular and useful softbill food but has some significant drawbacks.

Exoskeleton: the hard outer casing, called the exoskeleton, is made of chitin which is largely composed of cellulose. Most species, and especially young chicks, can find this difficult to digest since birds lack cellulase, the enzyme necessary to break down cellulose. (See Nutrition—carbohydrates and fats.)

Greatly overfeeding mealworms may therefore cause impaction (and ultimately death) as the chitin accumulates in the body. Mealworms should therefore be fed sparingly. And for omnivores, such as most starlings, that do not need much live food in a maintenance diet, 10 medium-sized mealworms a day is plenty.

Molted mealworms: as the mealworm grows it progresses through a series of molts, sloughing off its outer casing which is replaced by a fresh growth. At this stage its skin is white, soft and safe to eat, even for very young chicks, until the new (brown) casing is formed. Molted mealworms can be obtained by keeping the brown mealworms at room temperature and letting them grow.

Fat content: in practice the mealworm's high fat content tends to be more of a problem than its exoskeleton. Obesity can become life-threatening, especially for caged birds; and even when the softbill has a large area in which to exercise, mealworms must still be fed sparingly. What often happens is that an overabundance of mealworms leads to a bird that looks well-rounded and superficially healthy, while in fact it is malnourished and likely to get progressively worse. Ultimately death is the result.

Food for mealworms: the calcium content of mealworms tends to be low and this is worsened if the larvae have been fed on bran. The phytic acid in bran, known as a chelating agent, binds with calcium and prevents the bird's body from absorbing it. (See Nutrition—phytic acid.) Feeding mealworms poultry meal helps to overcome this problem, and being a nutritious food in itself, the meal enhances the overall food value of the mealworm. In Europe, live food nutrition has advanced to such a point that special diets and nutritional balancers are now available for mealworms and crickets. One of several insect food suppliers in the U.K. is The Mealworm Company Ltd, Unit 1, Universal Crescent, North Anston Trading Estate, Sheffield, S31 7JJ, U.K.

Propagating mealworms: at least 50 meal beetles (or mealworms that will turn into beetles) should be kept in a dry, well-ventilated container on about 2 in. (5 cm) of poultry meal. Provide slices of apple for moisture and keep the beetles at about 77°C (25°F). The meal beetle can fly, so cover the container with a perforated lid or a wire-mesh screen.

The adult beetles will lay their eggs in the poultry meal and then die—the beetles themselves are nutritious, and I like to mix pureed beetles in with the softbill foods. The eggs take six weeks to hatch; and at one month of age the larvae are more than 1 in. (2.4 cm) long and nearly ready to pupate.

The mealworms can be harvested at any time. If several colonies are established, at different stages of development, a range of mealworm sizes can be available. But they can be cannibalistic, so ensure that the larvae in each colony are of the same size.

Commercially produced mealworms: mealworms can be purchased fairly cheaply and are graded according to size.

Mini mealworms are ideal for chicks and small softbills

such as wrens, nuthatches, tits, warblers, bananaquits and sunbirds.

Standard mealworms are suitable for the vast majority of species.

Giant mealworms are best left to the large softbills such as crows and hornbills; and even then, only 2 or 3 should be fed per day.

American wax moth larvae, *Achroia melonella*

"Waxworms" are relished by almost all softbills and usually eaten in preference to mealworms. Their thin, soft skin makes them much safer as a rearing food; and like mealworms they can be harvested at any time during their two-month life cycle, whether 0.25 in. (0.6 cm) or 1 in. (2.4 cm) long. But waxworms are even more fattening than mealworms and their use must be moderated.

Propagating waxworms: commercially produced waxworms are usually irradiated to prevent them from spinning their cocoons. However, a commercial breeder or your local zoo will often be happy to supply a viable starter colony.

About 200 moths will be needed for a healthy colony which can be housed in a dry, well-ventilated container, similar to that used for mealworms. Their diet is highly nutritious: equal parts of wheatmeal and oatmeal (rolled oats) moistened with honey and water; or honey and glycerol. Drinking water is required, so provide a moist sponge or a very shallow dish. To stop the larvae from massing together and overheating, egg trays or rolls of thick paper can be put in the propagation box.

In the wild, wax moths will feed on the honeycomb of a dying beehive, cleaning it completely. A healthy beehive should be able to repel the moths fairly easily; nevertheless, if you live near an apiary, take the precaution of preventing any moths or larvae from escaping.

Crickets

Like mealworms these can be purchased according to size. The smallest and softest ones are the hatchlings, increasing in size to $\frac{1}{8}$ in., $\frac{1}{4}$ in., $\frac{1}{2}$ in. and 1 in. Crickets are less fattening than waxworms or mealworms.

Crickets can be purchased by mail order and do not die in transit as easily as mealworms or waxworms, even in warm weather. One thousand crickets can be purchased cheaply and maintained in an aquarium. Grass and cereal are adequate foods, but more nutritious for the crickets (and therefore more nutritious for your birds) are foods such as powdered primate pellets. Slices of potato are also beneficial. Provide drinking water in a shallow dish or moistened sponge. Cricket droppings accumulate very quickly and the aquarium will need regular cleaning, especially the water dish.

If keeping the crickets alive is too time consuming, just freeze the entire box on arrival. The frozen crickets can be included in the softbill diets, and are normally just as good and nutritious as live ones.

Propagating crickets: about 30 females should be removed from the main culture and put in an aquarium containing 4 in. (10 cm) of damp sand—the females can be recognized by the pointed tip on the abdomen which is used to lay the eggs in the sand. The eggs should be kept at about 81°F (27°C) and the humidity maintained by moistening the sand with a plant sprayer. The eggs take about 2 weeks to hatch with the young crickets completing their life cycle in only 6 weeks.

Locusts

Locusts have very similar requirements to crickets and can breed at 8 weeks of age. Adult locusts are much bigger than crickets and, because their life cycle is longer, tend to be more expensive. Consequently, these insects are not widely used, and in fact offer little that the cricket cannot provide.

Fruit flies, *Drosophila*

In the wild, nectivores such as hummingbirds and sunbirds may eat hundreds of small insects each day. Nowadays nectar foods take account of this by having a higher protein level than natural nectar. And so in the modern maintenance diet, fruit flies have become less important; but they are still vital during the run up to breeding and as a rearing food.

Propagating fruit flies: *drosophila* probably already exist in your bird room and are quite common in temperatures around 75°F

(24°C). Simply leave out a bucket of chopped fruits, and within days fruit flies will cloud around it. Sliced bananas are good to use since they do not mold as readily as other fruits and are less likely to promote diseases such as aspergillosis.

Starter culture: a more efficient and less smelly method of culturing flies is to use a culture medium obtainable from your pet store or live food supplier. Kits are sold containing test tubes and food. With only about 1 in. (2.4 cm) of food in each tube, a dozen flies rapidly multiply; and with several tubes, a continuous supply of *Drosophila* is assured.

In recent years wingless fruit flies have become available, and can be purchased as starter kits. They are ideal for smallish softbills that do not catch insects on the wing such as small tanagers, tits, bulbuls, *Chloropsis*, spiderhunters and nuthatches.

Whiteworms, *Enchytraeus*

At only about 0.5 in. (1.2 cm) in length, whiteworms are an ideal rearing food, although adult softbills do not like them as much as mealworms and waxworms.

Propagating whiteworms: purchasing a starter culture is difficult and the easiest option is to obtain a nucleus from your back yard. Find a damp, gloomy part of the garden and make a shallow hole about 6 in. (15 cm) in diameter. This will contain the bait which can be either a flour and water paste or bread soaked in water. Cover the hole with a piece of wood or slate, and replenish the food daily as increasing numbers of worms feast on it. Along with other worms, the small, hairlike whiteworms will be present and can be collected when there are enough. This represents the nucleus which can be divided into a number of starter colonies.

Fill several margarine containers with moist peat moss and press 1 or 2 holes into the peat of each container. In each hole deposit some bread soaked in water, and a portion of worms, so that the hole is half full. Keep the colony in complete darkness and at a temperature of about 70°F (21°C). The worms' food quickly becomes rancid, and excesses must be removed daily and replaced with fresh food. The worms are ready to harvest in about a month, but before using them, they should be thoroughly washed under running water to remove their, sometimes sour, food.

Maggots

Disease risk: maggots are arguably not an ideal food since they live on rotting meat and can bring botulism to your collection (see Ailments—botulism). However, sometimes they can satisfy a fussy parent in its search for acceptable live food.

The most important thing is to clean the maggots thoroughly before use. In unclean maggots, the ingested meat can be seen through the skin as a pink or black spot. On the very rare occasions I use maggots, I keep them on powdered chicken meal for at least 3 days until the meat has completely passed through them. Bran is also popular for cleaning maggots; but the phytic acid chelates calcium and other minerals making them unavailable to the bird. (See Nutrition.)

Propagating maggots: maggots can be purchased from fishing bait suppliers or they can be bred as easily as fruit flies. Any meat left outside in warm weather will become infested with them in only a few days. Hang the meat above a tray of the cleaning medium (powdered chicken meal) and collect the fallen maggots from the tray; start using them only when they are totally clean.

Fly maggots

To dispense flies into the aviary, put some maggots in an empty jar which has several small holes in the lid. As the maggots metamorphose into flies, they leave the jar and are eaten by the awaiting softbills.

Flies are especially valuable when birds such as flycatchers are rearing young. If chicks are present, I prefer to add handfuls of flies to the aviary to amply satisfy their needs. The flies alone are not especially nutritious and should only be used as part of a balanced diet. If they are for chicks, they must be sprinkled with a multivitamin and mineral supplement.

Ant pupae

Ant "eggs" are so nutritious that their collection is a must if ant nests are in the vicinity. They are relished by most birds and are especially important as a rearing food for very small softbills, chiefly insectivores.

Grass ant nests can be hard to find because they are hidden in lawns, but other ant nests are more conspicuous with craterlike mounds at the colony entrance. During the warmer months these nests are likely to contain many of the tiny white pupae, which can often be found buried only several centimeters below the surface.

Be careful when working on ant nests because most ants will bite, many will sting and a few can even eject a pungent-smelling secretion from their anus. It is best to wear boots and gloves, and it is also a good idea to tie down your pant cuffs.

To collect the pupae, lay a large piece of cloth beside the nest in direct sunlight. Fold the edges inward to make 2.5 in. (6 cm) flaps which are held up with stones and sticks. Remove the top layer of the nest and tip it onto the center of the cloth. Exposed to sunlight the pupae would quickly die, so they are taken by the ants to the dark protection under the flaps. Here the pupae are gathered into piles in an effort to rebuild the nest; they can be collected for immediate feeding or frozen for future use.

Earthworms

Earthworms are sold in small containers of peat moss and are often graded according to size. They are a good source of protein, but before they can be used as food, should be kept in the peat moss for several days. This allows the worms to void their guts of the potentially harmful decaying vegetation on which they feed. Thereafter, refrigeration will keep them fresh for about 3 weeks.

Earthworms are intermediate hosts for various parasites, and so on the very rare occasions I use them, my preference is to buy commercially produced worms. However, earthworms can be collected from your garden as follows: put some chopped vegetables in a secluded spot and cover them with a piece of wet burlap. Keep the cloth moist and simply dig up the worms that gather beneath it.

Although earthworms are not essential for an established softbill, they can be useful for a newly purchased or newly imported one. Thrushes and the like will easily eat a whole worm, but for species that may not be familiar with them, chopping the worm into short lengths works best.

I recently acclimated some bee eaters which arrived in a thin condition. To add variety to their diet, I chopped an earthworm into 0.5 in. (1.2 cm) lengths; and after several days of eating their favorite foods, the bee eaters began to eat the worm pieces.

Mice

Mice are commercially produced and sold in three stages of development.

Adults   are suitable for toucans, hornbills, large shrikes and large kingfishers; and can be fed whole or chopped, depending on the size of the bird.

"Fuzzies"   are younger mice with the first growth of velvetlike fur. They are suitable for kingfishers, jays, magpies, certain starlings, and African and Asian barbets; and should be chopped to suit the softbill.

"Pinkies"   are newborn mice. Small, naked and soft, they are full of nutrition and can be included in the diet of all meat-eating species. Very finely sliced they are excellent in the diets of difficult softbills, such as bee eaters; and they are equally good as a hand-rearing food for all softbill chicks (except nectivores) from about day 6—freezing the pinkies makes it easier to finely slice them.

Softbill Diets

If you already enjoy success with a particular diet, do not change it. But contained in this section are suggested recipes that have been tried and tested over several years, every one with a consistent record of breeding success. To enable you to make a diet with local ingredients, alternatives are given for foods that may not be available worldwide.

Diets for omnivores

For dietary purposes, omnivores can be divided into 2 broad groups:

A) meat-biased—species that need more meat or insects;
B) fruit-biased—species that need more fruit.

Diet A for meat-biased omnivores: barbets (Asian and African), crows, drongos, jays, laughing thrushes, magpies, marshbirds, mockingbirds, mynahs, oropendolas, Pekin robin, silver-eared mesia, sivas, starlings, tree pies and the troupial.

Diet: 45 percent fruit, 37 percent proprietary softbill pellets, 10 percent chopped, hard-boiled egg, 5 percent live food, 3 percent vegetables and greens.

Live food is not normally essential in a maintenance diet, but is vital during the breeding season. Fed in moderation, meats such as chopped pinkie mice or lean hamburger can help bring the meat-biased omnivores into breeding condition.

Diet B for fruit-biased omnivores: barbets (South American), birds of paradise, bulbuls, *Chloropsis*, cotingas such as cocks of the rock, fairy bluebirds, honeyeaters, ioras, lesser green broadbill, manakins, tanagers including euphonias and chlorophonias, and toucans.

Diet: 50 percent fruit, 33 percent proprietary softbill pellets, 10 percent chopped, hard-boiled egg, 5 percent vegetables and greens, 2 percent live food.

Chloropsis, honeyeaters and ioras also need a small dish of nectar with a pellet (such as a primate pellet) floating in it; the nectar can simply be sugar water, but lory or hummingbird nectar is far better (see Diet D). And to a lesser extent, tanagers, fairy bluebirds and manakins also benefit from nectar.

Toucans and South American barbets are primarily fruit eaters; but lean hamburger or pinkie mice are beneficial in moderation, especially to help achieve breeding condition.

Diet preparation for diet A and diet B: the fruits and vegetables should be diced into cubes of between 0.25 in. (0.6 cm) and 0.5 in. (1.2 cm). If offered chunks or slices most softbills will still be able to eat them; but in the wild, species such as toucans, hornbills, touracos and fruit pigeons and doves swallow berries whole, and are less able to break up their food. Try to provide pieces that can be picked up and swallowed easily.

The finished diet should be loose and moist to the touch. Avoid large amounts of fruit juice, or the mixture will become an inedible sludge.

The ingredients can be offered either as a mixture or in separate piles (cafeteria style). Some very successful aviculturists offer food separately; but this type of feeding may encourage birds to eat only their favorite foods and not the range necessary for optimum health. My preference is to mix the ingredients together to ensure a balanced intake.

Diet C for frugivores: fruit doves and pigeons, mousebirds, touracos and waxwings.

In practice, frugivores do well on a diet very similar to the fruit-biased omnivore diet B. But it is important to separate the frugivores into their own group, because for long-term health they tend to need a lower protein intake. (See Nutrition—protien requirements.)

Diet: 55 percent fruit, 30 percent proprietary softbill pellets, 10 percent chopped, hard-boiled egg, 5 percent vegetables and greens.

Diet preparation is the same as that described in the omnivore section.

Diets for nectivores

Diet D for hummingbirds: there are a number of hummingbird nectars available. An excellent one that has produced good breeding results is Nektar-Plus (distributed by Nekton U.S.A., Inc., Clearwater, Florida). This is a complete maintenance diet for which large amounts of fruit flies are not essential; but some fruit flies are highly beneficial and a requisite for breeding. (See Live Food—fruit flies.)

The nectar comes as a powder which is mixed with water according to the manufacturer's instructions, and offered in test-tube-like feeders. These are available in glass or plastic, and have a small, red feeding spout at the bottom.

Hummingbirds can be quite pugnacious and are likely to chase each other from time to time. Provide at least one feeder per bird, so that if a hummingbird is chased, it is never very far from food. For newly assembled groups, even more feeders will be needed until the birds settle down and establish rough territories.

Certain hummingbirds are famous for their ability to slow their heart rate and reduce their body temperature, going into a coma-like state (called noctivation or torpor) at the end of each day. In the wild, this is an important mechanism for saving energy. But in captivity it is not normal to go into a state of torpor and may well indicate illness or substandard food; in fact the need for torpidity is associated with the lack of food rather than cold nights. The use of a night light is therefore important to allow continuous feeding.

Diet E for sunbirds and spiderhunters: a proprietary hummingbird nectar is ideal for these softbills. Offer the nectar and primate pellet or sponge cake, in an open dish. But be careful with newly purchased or imported specimens, which may be weak or sick. They can easily fall in the nectar and drown, or mistake it for a bath. Protect such birds by placing a piece of wire mesh over the dish.

Diet: in one dish, 50 percent nectar, 50 percent sponge cake, bread or primate pellet. In a separate dish, finely chopped fruits with fine grade insectivore diet G sprinkled over them; include small mealworms, small waxworms and $1/4$ in. crickets. Fruit flies (for the sunbirds) and fly maggots (for the spiderhunters) complete a healthy diet.

Diet F for other nectivores: bananaquit, *Dacnis*, honeycreepers (sugarbirds), yuhinas and white eyes require food similar to diet E, but presented slightly differently.

Diet: in one dish, 50 percent nectar, 25 percent fruit, 25 percent sponge cake, bread or primate pellet. In a separate dish, fine grade insectivore diet G with small mealworms, small waxworms and $1/4$ in. crickets. Supply fruit flies and fly maggots.

Diets for insectivores

Diet G for standard insectivores: bluethroat, bush robins, chats, cuckoos, flycatchers, hoopoe (common), minivets, niltavas, nuthatches, parrotbills, pittas, robins, rubythroat, redstarts, shamas, tits, tit babblers, treecreepers, wagtails, warblers, wallcreepers, woodpeckers, wrens and wren babblers.

In the U.K., the "powdered, proprietary softbill pellets" and "powdered trout chow" can be replaced by Prosecto or Claus Fat Food-type IV (blue).

Diet: 50 percent powdered proprietary softbill pellets, 15 percent finely chopped, hard-boiled egg, 10 percent powdered trout chow, 10 percent live food, 9 percent pureed apple, 6 percent tofu.

In the wild, fruits and berries are often eaten by some insectivores, although in captivity I have not found them to be popular. Chopped fruits alone are not very nutritious, so if they are used, increase their food value with a multivitamin and mineral supplement.

Diet preparation: the key to making a diet for the tiny insectivores is to ensure that the softbill pellets and trout chow are a powder. The trout chow can be purchased as a powder but you will probably have to break up the softbill pellets yourself in a food processor. Tropical Bits are a notable exception that do not have to be powdered, since they are tiny enough even for the smallest insectivores, such as tits and nuthatches. (See Proprietary Softbill Pellets.)

In their dry state these ingredients are useless and need to be moistened to be made palatable. The tofu and pureed apple will provide much of the necessary moisture, and if more is needed, tap water or fruit juice can be added.

Mix the ingredients by squeezing them together, and break up any lumps to arrive at a very fine consistency. The dry powders should now be moist while still being crumbly.

Diet H for difficult insectivores: bee eaters, Asian and African trogons, and paradise, monarch, fantail and wattle-eye flycatchers.

Once acclimated, the vast majority of insectivores are relatively easy to maintain on diet G. But certain species or specimens need diet H, which can be used, along with the meating-off techniques, to acclimate even the most difficult birds. See meating-off.

In the U.K., Prosecto or Claus softbill food could be used in place of the powdered softbill pellet and trout chow, as in diet G. But my preference is not to use them because they do not tend to stick as well to the live food, pinkies, etc., and the birds therefore do not receive such good all-round nutrition.

Diet: 40 percent powdered proprietary softbill pellets, 20 percent live food, 9 percent pureed apple, 9 percent finely chopped, hard-boiled egg, 8 percent powdered trout chow, 7 percent tofu, 5 percent finely sliced pinkies (1 mm thick), 2 percent chopped earthworms.

Diet preparation: mix the powdered softbill pellets, powdered trout chow, pureed apple and tofu together as described in diet G. The mixture should be of a fine consistency and will fill about half of the food dish. The remaining ingredients (live food, egg, sliced pinkies and earthworms) lay on top of this mixture and stimulate feeding by being clearly visible. However, consumption of the powdered softbill pellets and trout chow is the key to long-term success, and must be brought about by various methods as described in meating-off. (See photo section beginning on page 129.)

Meating-off

This is the process of converting a bird from its natural diet to an artificial one, and is especially useful when acclimating difficult insectivores such as bee eaters and certain trogons.

In the wild, insectivores' nutritional requirements are met by a very wide variety of insects, along with the equally varied diets those insects live on. In captivity, we cannot provide such a huge range of foods; so over the years artificial diets have been made, incorporating live food, but largely consisting of man-made ingredients. The commercially available mealworms, waxworms and crickets do not provide a balanced diet and ultimately lead to malnutrition. To encourage the insectivore onto a more balanced (artificial) diet is therefore as urgent as it is essential.

How to meat-off: the live food should be dipped in a stiff nectar or honey solution and rolled in the powdered softbill pellets—do not suffocate the insects since their movement is needed to stimulate feeding. And with the powders now sticking to the insects, the birds will receive a nutritious food with every mouthful. A taste for the artificial ingredients will eventually be developed and the birds' reliance on live food diminished. The finely chopped, hard-boiled egg is also important, and eaten by most insectivores, even when newly imported.

The time taken to meat-off a bird will vary, but the process can be quickened if a "teacher" bird is present. This is an established softbill of the same or similar species that is used to the captive diet, and can teach the newcomer by example.

Supplements: these can be valuable for difficult insectivores, primarily if the birds are reluctant to eat the artificial foods. Nekton Tonic I is a supplement designed for insectivores and available from Nekton U.S.A. Inc., Clearwater, Florida. I sprinkle this over the diet twice a week if an insectivore (usually a bee eater) is not yet eating the full range of nutritious foods. And even when fully acclimated and established, very difficult insectivores still benefit from Nekton Tonic I twice a week.

But remember, if a softbill is eating the appropriate amounts of a proprietary softbill pellet, dietary supplements are unlikely to be necessary in a maintenance diet, and may lead to an overabundance of certain vitamins and minerals, with potentially harmful results.

Where to position the food dish: the difficult insectivores are generally birds that catch food on the wing, and are unwilling to use a food dish on the floor (unless the dish is on the floor of a cage that is raised several feet above the ground). Position the food at least 3' (90 cm) above the ground, and in an open area, so that birds like bee eaters and kingfishers can feed by hovering. Shier birds will get much of their food by hovering, but once established, will perch on and in the dish.

Diet I for carnivores: ground hornbills, kookaburras and roadrunners.

Diet: 30 percent Bird of Prey Diet, 30 percent adult mice or day-old chicks, 25 percent powdered, proprietary softbill pellets, 10 percent soaked dog or cat chow, 5 percent large mealworms or crickets. Bird of Prey diet is a proprietary processed meat available in the United States and commonly used by zoos. It is packed by Central Nebraska Packing Inc., North Platte, Nebraska. An acceptable equivalent is ground lean beef or turkey. Kookaburras and most other kingfishers may also eat small fish.

Diet preparation: the powdered softbill pellets and the soaked chow are mixed into the Bird of Prey Diet. The impregnated meat can then be offered in small balls alongside the mice and insects. Small mice with bodies about 2 in. (5 cm) long do not need to be chopped for birds of kookaburra size. But if day-old chicks are used they will need to be halved or quartered for all but the largest, hornbill-sized, carnivores—this is easier if the mice are semifrozen.

Diet J for rails: coots, crakes, gallinules, rails and water hens.

Diet: 35 percent powdered proprietary softbill pellets, 20 percent Bird of Prey Diet (see Diet I) or lean hamburger, 15 percent chopped, hard-boiled egg, 18 percent soaked dog or cat chow, 10 percent live food, 2 percent canary seed.

Diet preparation: all should be mixed together, breaking the ingredients into small pieces. The finished diet must be fairly moist, while remaining crumbly. If it is too dry, add water and mix thoroughly.

Diet K for shore birds: avocets, curlews, dotterels, dowitchers, godwits, jacanas, knots, lapwings, oystercatchers, phalaropes, plovers, redshanks, sandpipers, sandplovers, snipes, stilts, stints and woodcocks.

Diet: 38 percent powdered, proprietary softbill pellets, 20 percent chopped, hard-boiled egg, 15 percent soaked dog or cat chow, 15 percent Bird of Prey Diet (see Diet I) or lean hamburger, 12 percent live food including chopped earthworms.

Diet preparation: mix all of the ingredients together. The meat pieces should be very small and it may be necessary to roll them into individual balls. The entire diet should comprise loose, moist and small food pieces that these fine-billed birds can easily pick up.

7

Nutrition

Proteins, Fats and Carbohydrates

Proteins and amino acids

Proteins are built of amino acids and are essential for a healthy body, making up the muscles, blood, feathers and skin. They come in many shapes and sizes, and the most familiar ones are enzymes, antibodies and hormones. Enzymes control the chemical reactions of metabolism; antibodies help fight infection; and hormones, such as adrenalin, assist in regulating body systems.

The body's structural materials are made of fibrous proteins: actin and myosin are found in muscle; collagen forms the body's ligaments and keratin makes up the skin, claws and feathers.

Of the many amino acids, 10 are essential for all vertebrates, and for certain species additional amino acids are also necessary. The 10 essential acids are arginine, histidine, leucine, isoleucine, lysine, methionine, phenylalanine, threonine, tryptophan and valine. Glutamic acid, glycine and proline may also be important in a softbill diet since they are required for optimal growth in chickens.

The essential amino acids must be present in a bird's diet because they cannot be synthesized by the body to adequately meet metabolic needs. In their absence, a diet will be deficient even if the percentage of protein may appear acceptable. Food should provide the essential amino acids in a balanced form; specifically, the quality of a particular protein source can be assessed by its amino acid profile (or content), which should be similar to that of the bird's body.

Protein requirements

The entire body requires proteins. In a normal bird about 5 percent of body proteins are replaced daily; injury and activity increase the rate of turnover. A balanced diet should contain both animal and vegetable proteins. The amount consumed depends on whether the bird eats primarily fruits, insects, nectar or meat.

Studies have shown that the live foods commonly used in captivity (crickets, mealworms and waxworms) contain approximately 20 percent protein. And in practice, insectivores are long lived and successful breeders when fed a diet of 20 to 25 percent protein, as are carnivores.

Omnivores thrive on slightly lower protein levels of 15 to 20 percent since lower protein foods such as fruits and leaves form the foundation of many of their diets. But in the run-up to the breeding season, the consumption of protein increases as omnivores begin to feast on the seasonal abundance of insects.

And while the pure frugivores do equally well on many omnivore diets, protein levels should be moderated to avoid renal damage and perhaps even excessive aggression.

Although captive omnivores are often given live food year-round, in the presence of a good diet, they do not especially need it, unless rearing chicks or being stimulated in the hope of breeding. Indeed an excess of live food, chiefly mealworms and waxworms, can cause life-threatening obesity and/or malnutrition, as the nutritionally better parts of the diet are permanently ignored.

Carbohydrates and fats

These deliver the calories a body needs for energy and warmth. Carbohydrates are primary energy units and are classified as soluble or insoluble. Nutritionally, the soluble carbohydrates are the most significant and come in the form of sugars and starches. These are what the body uses now while fats represent the main means of storing energy.

The major part of many softbill diets is fruit. Although a relatively poor source of certain vitamins and minerals, fruit does contain nature's sugar, fructose, from which the body can make carbohydrates. These are fairly quickly burned up by physical activity while an excess, in the form of glycogen, can be stored in the liver and used whenever and wherever the body needs it. If the body's intake of carbohydrates is not fully used, an excess of starches will tend to create fat accumulations.

A healthy bird should always have some body fat as a precautionary measure. This will help cushion body organs and protect the bird from the cold: when oxidized, fats produce at least twice the energy of carbohydrates or proteins. In the wild, fats also provide the energy necessary for migration.

Key components of fat are called fatty acids and, like amino acids, they must be present in a bird's diet. Linoleic and linolenic acids are essential fatty acids. Arachidonic acid is sometimes considered essential, but can be synthesized from linoleic acid. Essential fatty acids are the precursors of prostaglandins which have many hormonelike effects such as inducing lower blood pressure and smoothing muscle operation.

Body Condition Index

Whenever a bird is handled, its general body condition can be assessed by feeling the amount of breast muscle. The Body Condition Index (BCI) can then used to describe the amount of flesh on the keel.

I Emaciated (Scant flesh on keel)
II Thin (Prominent keel)
III Normal (Well-padded keel)
IV Fat (Keel is a depression on the breast)
V Obese (Abundant flesh—keel cannot be felt)

Dietary fiber

The insoluble carbohydrates, such as lignin and cellulose, are better known as dietary fiber. They are complex carbohydrates that are partially or completely indigestible because birds lack cellulase, the enzyme necessary to break down cellulose. Although of no direct nutritional value, these carbohydrates can affect digestion.

Many birds possess a pair of dead-end sacs or tubes called the caeca. They are located toward the posterior end of the intestine and vary widely in size, being very small or even nonexistent in some families. Their main function is to absorb water and digested nutrients, and especially cellulose that has been bacterially decomposed. Dietary fiber (insoluble carbohydrates) regulates the transit time of food through the gastrointestinal tract and therefore it regulates microbial digestion in the caeca. Fiber also influences gut vitamin synthesis and gut flora populations.

Cellulose is the main component of chitin which makes up the skin and exoskeleton of insects. Hard-bodied insects, particularly mealworms, should therefore be fed sparingly since they can be difficult to digest, especially for chicks. A few softbills, however, experience no such problems. Bee eaters kill quite large insects by beating them against a perch, before swallowing them whole. The indigestible residue is then regurgitated in the form of a pellet, similar to what an owl or hawk does, a process that seems to be assisted by the bird whacking its beak against the perch. Kingfishers also produce pellets in a similar way.

Drinking and Bathing Water

Often overlooked as a nutrient, water makes up more than half of a bird's body. Consumption depends on environmental factors, physical activity and diet, with the dry and highly nutritious pelleted foods tending to heighten a bird's thirst. Although fruits and insects provide much moisture, access to fresh drinking water is essential for most species, and should not be denied for more than an hour, especially in hot weather. However, veterinarians often require food and water to be withheld prior to surgery. Healthy softbills of starling size and larger may go without water when shipped in temperatures not exceeding about 75°F (24°C) on journeys of less than 6 hours.

Bathing water is also necessary for softbills to maintain peak condition, especially for birds, such as hummingbirds, that rely entirely on their flying ability for their survival. The depth of water depends on the species, for very small or sick birds, 0.5 in. (1.2 cm) is best.

The uropygial (preen) gland is located at the base of the tail and secretes an oil that is spread over the feathers during preening. This waterproofs the plumage, making it more durable and possibly helping to prevent skin infections. Most birds bathe regularly, preen and maintain a waterproofed plumage. But if bathing water has not been available or has not been used, the natural waterproofing will be diminished or lost.

This is especially dangerous if birds are moved outdoors and expected to withstand an occasional shower of rain; or if they are moved to an aviary with large pools and fast-flowing streams. Without waterproofing they will get soaked to the skin and will not be able to fly until their feathers have dried—such birds will need to be kept warm to avoid becoming chilled.

Waterproofing and general feather quality can be maintained by using a plant sprayer or, for large hornbill-sized birds, a hose with a fine spray nozzle. For breeding aviaries, a misting system is highly beneficial, encouraging many birds to bathe much more frequently than they otherwise would. (See Breeding Stimuli—rain.)

Vitamins and Minerals

With so many high quality vitamin and mineral supplements available, this section may seem to be somewhat redundant. But vitamin and mineral deficiencies still occur in modern collections and recognizing them is therefore important. Even the so-called complete proprietary diets are not perfect, since few are actually researched for optimum balance. Instead, most softbill diets are based on personal experience and are extrapolated from known species such as chickens.

Thin-shelled eggs, poor plumage, eye problems, nervous disorders such as "star gazing" and the fungal infection *Candida* can all be linked to specific mineral or vitamin deficiencies. The following sections are intended to show how vital a nutritionally balanced diet is and how pertinent it is to breeding success. Source foods are given for each vitamin and mineral. These are listed in rough order of potency, beginning with the best source.

Vitamins

The study of vitamins began with Drs. Grijns and Eyckman, as they discovered a property in rice hulls that protected people from beri-

beri. That property was isolated to a substance that was later called a vitamin, specifically vitamin B. We now know that substance as the vitamin B complex, made up of 12 substances, the most familiar being B_1, B_2, B_6 and B_{12}.

Vitamins are complex, organic molecules. They comprise the elements hydrogen, oxygen and carbon, and often nitrogen, sometimes including minerals like sulfur and phosphorus. Their functions are many, the most important being the maintenance of cells and the operation of various organs.

Most of the B vitamins function as coenzymes, acting as the body's ignition keys and regulators. Other vitamins, called antioxidants, protect key molecules from damage, while others still, act as hormones controlling growth, metabolic functions and even sexuality.

Fat soluble and water soluble

Vitamins A, D, E and K are fat soluble, being found in fatty substances and generally stored in the bodies of animals. These can amass in the body to the point of being toxic and are not removed via the urine. Instead, their loss is in bile pigments which are recycled and depleted slowly. Other vitamins, however, cannot be stored in the body and so must be constantly provided by food: these are water soluble and their excesses can be removed through the urine. Such vitamins are: B_1, B_2, B_3, B_6, B_{12} and C as well as folic acid and choline.

Vitamin A

Vitamin A travels through the blood stream, on a protein, to reach every cell in the body. Proteins of sufficient quality and quantity must therefore be present otherwise the vitamin cannot be utilized.

Because an overdose of this fat-soluble vitamin can be toxic, adding its precursor, carotene, to a diet may be safer. A body can then manufacture the vitamin according to its needs, rather than having to absorb whatever amount is present in the food.

Vitamin A is necessary for the growth of new tissue and its absence will result in the slow growth or death of young birds. Generally the vitamin promotes healthy skin and bones, with the upper layer of the skin (epithelium) affected in vitamin-deficient specimens. The skin cells enlarge, die quickly and form areas of flaky accumulations. Vitamin A is mostly stored in the liver with some in the kidneys: a deficiency will cause gout as the kidneys become unable to remove uric acid. Resistance to infection is also lowered and fertility is sharply reduced, leading ultimately to impotence.

Eye infections, and in severe cases blindness, can also be caused by a deficiency. *Candida albicans* is a fungal infection of the mouth and upper digestive tract. It is due to reduced resistance in damaged or defective skin layers and can sometimes be attributed to a vitamin A deficiency. In such cases a brief, high dose of the vitamin may be beneficial. Check with your veterinarian. (See also Ailments.)

Source of vitamin A: liver, cod liver oil, peanuts, milk and eggs.

Source of carotenes: red, yellow and orange vegetables, such as carrots, sweet potato, corn, tomatoes, paprika and papaya; and greens.

Vitamin B_1 (Thiamine)

Thiamine aids in carbohydrate metabolism and is especially important for a healthy nervous system. Deficiencies can cause weak legs and tail, or central nervous system problems such as head tilt and star gazing. A bird's appetite can also be affected and is sometimes accompanied by digestive problems with loose or poor quality droppings.

Source: brewer's yeast, corn, rice, eggs, potatoes, green vegetables particularly peas and beans; and avocados—see also vitamin E for warning.

Vitamin B_2 (Riboflavin)

Although B_2 is only required in small amounts, it is essential for the basic cellular metabolism of glucose. In the body, riboflavin is unlikely to become toxic since it is rapidly lost in urine. High doses turn the urates bright yellow which may be misinterpreted as liver disease.

Riboflavin promotes healthy skin, feathers and claws as well as encouraging a normal appetite and a good digestion. It is especially important for young birds, although all will suffer in its absence, experiencing eye problems and varying degrees of paralysis.

Source: brewer's yeast, liver, fish, eggs, cheese, corn and green vegetables.

Vitamin B_3 (Niacin)

Niacin is essential for normal breeding, a healthy metabolism and skin quality. Deficiencies lead to very poor plumage, reduced growth, poor appetite, sore eyes and scaly dermatitis, predominantly on the legs and corners of the beak.

Source: brewer's yeast, peanuts, corn, rice, potatoes, green vegetables; and avocados—see also vitamin E for warning.

Vitamin B_6 (Pyridoxine)

Vitamin B_6 aids in the production of red blood cells and antibodies while controlling the metabolism in the liver and nerves. Deficiencies can cause poor feathering and depressed growth with a general loss of weight, appetite and breeding performance.

Source: brewer's yeast, liver, peanuts, blackstrap molasses, rice, bananas, corn, eggs and green vegetables; and avocados—see also vitamin E for warning.

Vitamin B_{12} (Cobalamin)

The main commercial form of cobalamin is cyanocobalamin. It is important for healthy intestinal bacteria (flora) and in its absence, digestion is affected. The quality of egg hatches can suffer as embryos die following only partial development. Chicks may exhibit poor feathering, liver damage and slow growth. Deficiencies can also cause nerve damage, anemia and bone deformities, and blood cell production can be affected.

"Star gazing" describes a condition where the bird looks upward far more often than is normal while moving its head around jerkily. A vitamin deficiency is not necessarily the cause, but when it is, a B_{12} injection or food supplement can be very effective.

Source: seafoods, liver, eggs, cheese, milk and brewer's yeast.

Folic acid

Folic acid is also one of the B vitamins. It is necessary for the production of red blood cells and generally in the body's use of proteins. Deficiencies can cause anemia and may impair normal feather and body growth. With anemia comes exhaustion. An affected bird will weaken rapidly, tending to sit on the floor, perhaps suffering leg pains. Deficiencies are unlikely, however, since folic acid is widespread in nature.

Source: brewer's yeast, liver, peanuts, soybeans, rice, corn, eggs, beans, beets and spinach.

Choline

Choline helps in functions of the nervous system along with the metabolizing of fats and cholesterol. It is involved in normal liver and kidney processes and a deficiency can cause fats to accumulate in the liver until the cirrhosis is irreversible.

Source: brewer's yeast, peanuts, beans, peas, eggs, rice and potatoes.

Vitamin C (Ascorbic acid)

Vitamin C assists in the formation of collagen, a strong yet flexible material used in parts of the body where bone would be too rigid. Generally the vitamin helps to fight infection and heal injuries as well as helping to produce red blood cells.

Most birds can synthesize vitamin C (from glucose) themselves. However, the red-vented bulbul and perhaps some toucans cannot. Since their natural diet contains sufficient vitamin C, there has been no pressure on them to produce the acid themselves. And it would be reasonable to assume that other avian species are also unable to synthesize it. Such birds must receive the vitamin in their food, on almost a daily basis, since it is not adequately stored in body tissues.

Source: guavas, black currants, strawberries, persimmons, citrus fruits, tomatoes and green vegetables.

Vitamin D_3

Unlike mammals, birds cannot utilize D_2 so they must have D_3 for good health. When exposed to the sun's ultraviolet rays the provitamin (7-dehydrocholesterol) is synthesized. At the bird's skin it is converted to D_3 and absorbed.

Glass filters out the beneficial wavelengths of sunlight and so it can be helpful to open some of the bird room windows during summer. Full-spectrum Vitalites™ also produce the ultraviolet wavelengths needed for synthesis, but the bird must be within about 3 ft. (0.9 m) of them to receive the full benefit.

Vitamin D_3 regulates the body's calcium and phosphorus levels, controlling the amount absorbed by the intestine while acting on the kidneys to affect the amount excreted from the body. Since it facilitates calcium absorption, D_3 is essential in preventing rickets, soft-shelled eggs, egg binding, poor growth, paralysis and malformed bones. "Angel wing" may also be partly caused by a D_3 deficiency.

Dietary excess of vitamin D_3 can cause a demineralized and weakened skeleton, and hypercalcemia: calcium deposition in the heart, kidneys, arteries and other tissues causing irreversible damage.

Source: direct sunlight, cod liver oil, egg yolk and cheeses.

Vitamin E

Contrary to popular belief there is little evidence that increased levels of vitamin E can improve fertility. A deficiency, however, can reduce fertility and may lead to sterility.

Principally, vitamin E acts as an antioxidant, protecting cell membranes as well as helping to regenerate damaged tissue. Deficiencies can lead to a wasting away of muscles, edema and enlarged glands.

Avocados are very high in vitamin E and can be toxic to some birds; they are also particularly high in lipids (fatty substances such as fats and oils). If avocados are used, they should comprise no more than about 5 percent of a softbill diet. For parrots, avocados are even more dangerous and should not be fed at all.

Source: avocados, green vegetables, fish, corn and dried milk.

Vitamin K

From the Danish word *koagulate*, vitamin K is essential for the normal clotting of blood. Without it, clotting is slow, bruising is made easier and internal bleeding becomes more likely. Vitamin K is synthesized by the gut flora and is necessary for a healthy liver.

Source: green vegetables, eggs, milk, liver, carrots and fish meal.

Minerals

Minerals are inorganic elements; they are atoms as opposed to molecular compounds such as vitamins. The body requires minerals for countless vital functions such as building materials and as components of vitamins. The skeleton depends largely on minerals for its structure, tissues grow using minerals, the acid/alkali balance of blood is controlled by them, as is the transportation of oxygen throughout the body, the manufacture of red blood corpuscles and numerous other functions.

Some vitamins accumulate in the body while others are passed out in the urine and feces. All minerals, however, are water soluble and are therefore subject to fecal loss.

The absorption and utilization of minerals are regulated by hormones, body chemistry, and counterbalance and competition effects with other minerals. Oversupplementation must therefore be guarded against, since an excess of one mineral can affect the functioning of another, with potentially harmful results.

Most animals have special mechanisms to collect and store minerals; some are very efficient where certain minerals are typically rare in a native habitat. For example, most toucans are susceptible to iron-storage poisoning. Generally, members of this family should have diets low in iron.

Copper

Copper facilitates the absorption of iron in the intestines. It also helps in the production of hemoglobin and is essential for healthy blood. A deficiency can cause anemia and consequently feathers may become discolored.

Source: brewer's yeast, molasses, liver, oysters, mussels, honey, bananas, rice; and avocados—see vitamin E for warning.

Calcium

Bones are substantially calcium phosphate; calcium is therefore a prerequisite for the development and growth of a healthy skeleton. It is also used to help blood clot and in the manufacture of egg shell, along with the correct functioning of the heart, muscles and nervous system.

Deficiencies can cause muscle weakness, brittle or rubbery bones, or poor bone growth. Chicks are especially susceptible to such disorders so adding a calcium (and vitamin D_3) supplement to the rearing food is highly recommended. This is particularly so for young insectivores which seem to develop rickets more easily than other softbills. (See also Ailments—rickets.)

Source: dicalcium phosphate, calcium carbonate, bone meal, powdered milk, cheese and eggs.

Phosphorus

It is important that the body does not have a great surplus of phosphorus: this will be excreted in the form of calcium phosphate, dragging calcium from the body and potentially causing a calcium deficiency. A surplus may also result in excessive levels of phosphorus being deposited in bone making the skeleton weak. Consequently, in a healthy body the calcium:phosphorus ratio must be in equilibrium at approximately 2:1.

Calcium and phosphorus make up the building blocks of bone. Phosphorus also contributes to the growth and renewal of cells and its deficiency can cause slow tissue healing, poor bone growth and bone disease.

Source: dicalcium phosphate, bone meal, brewer's yeast, peanuts, eggs and vegetables.

Chlorine and sodium

These minerals are required to maintain the correct acid/alkali balance of the blood while also helping to regulate the body's fluids. Deficiencies of either mineral can cause dehydration with inadequate levels of chlorine also leading to abnormal digestion, since in a healthy body it produces stomach acids.

Source of chlorine: salt, dairy products, eggs, carrots, molasses and meat and fish products.

Source of sodium: salt, bone meal, powdered milk, fish meal and eggs.

Potassium

Deficiencies can be caused by an excess of sodium or a substantial loss of body fluids, such as in diarrhea. If left unremedied, a loss of potassium can interfere with normal growth and the development of a healthy skeleton, especially in young birds. General muscle weakness can also be experienced, leading to emaciation and ultimately death. In addition, potassium is involved in the regulation of the body's pH and energy balance.

Source: molasses, brewer's yeast, soybean products, vegetables and fruits, especially bananas; and avocados—see also vitamin E for warning.

Iodine

Iodine serves only one, but very important purpose. Entering the thyroid glands it becomes part of the hormone thyroxin which regulates the body's metabolism.

An iodine deficiency can lead to the condition known as goiter. The thyroid glands become enlarged and the resultant pressure on the windpipe often leads to noisy breathing. Vomiting may also occur although such problems are rare in softbills with the few occurrences more likely among seed-eaters, since seed is frequently low in iodine.

Moderate excesses of dietary iodine are usually efficiently excreted from the body. But prolonged consumption of excessive iodine causes reduced iodine uptake by the thyroid, leading to a disrupted metabolism and goitrogenic effects.

Certain foods contain a substance called thio-oxazidone which actually prevents iodine absorption, a property neutralized by cooking. Such foods include turnips, beets, spinach, cabbage, lettuce and broccoli.

Source: dried whey, iodized salt, seafood, cod liver oil, eggs, cheese, brewer's yeast and molasses.

Iron

This is a fundamental part of perhaps the body's most important protein, hemoglobin. Hemoglobin is what blood owes its color to, but more importantly it is the molecule that carries oxygen from the lungs to the rest of the entire body.

In iron-deficient birds, hemoglobin production falls, leading to iron-deficiency anemia. As a result, the whole body suffers from fatigue, general muscle weakness and pale mucous membranes. Excesses are also dangerous because they interfere with the body's use of vitamin D, causing disruptions to bone growth. In addition, iron-storage disease can affect most softbills, manifesting itself in a distended abdomen, liver disease and a progressive inability to fly. (See Ailments—iron-storage disease.)

Source: bone meal, fish and meat meals, calcium carbonate, brewer's yeast, egg yolk, snails, green vegetables and soybeans.

Magnesium

Magnesium is necessary for metabolizing carbohydrates and exists in bone, tissue and egg shell. A deficiency can be caused by an excess of calcium, since together the two minerals are transported through the blood on the protein albumen. Because they must share this transport, it is important that magnesium and calcium are roughly in equilibrium.

Magnesium activates most of the enzymes that use B_1, B_2 and B_6 as coenzymes. Deficiencies of these vitamins are therefore similar to a deficiency of magnesium and can result in impaired bone development, poor plumage and incoordination. Dietary excess of magnesium can cause diarrhea, decreased egg production and thin-shelled eggs.

Source: bone meal, brewer's yeast, kelp, snails, soybeans, rice, fruits and vegetables.

Manganese

Manganese is very important in the growth of feathers, the quality of egg production and the normal development of young birds. It is also necessary for the regeneration of blood and bone with deficiencies leading to bone disease, anemia, slow development of embryos, an unhealthy metabolism and "angel wing."

Source: dicalcium phosphate, calcium carbonate, soy products, tea leaves, green vegetables, rice and snails.

Zinc

A number of enzymes require zinc to function properly and the body also needs it to help with healing processes. Zinc is necessary for reproduction, healthy bone, the formation of egg shell and the normal growth of young birds. A deficiency disrupts the metabolism, slows growth, affects feather quality and may diminish feather pigment. Zinc requirements are increased with calcium added to the diet.

Source: fish, meat, bone and soybean meal, eggs, corn and green vegetables.

Mineral Inhibitors

Oxalic acid

This is an organic acid that binds calcium and other trace elements, preventing the body from using them. Oxalic acid is found in high levels in spinach; and in lower levels in peas, beets, carrots, lettuce, turnips and berries. In practice, all of these foods are safe provided they are part of a balanced intake. But spinach should be used more carefully and kept below about 5 percent (by volume) of the diet.

Phytic acid

This is a complex of phosphoric acid and sugar which effectively chelates minerals such as iron, zinc and calcium, making them unavailable to the body. Phytic acid is commonly found in legumes, nuts and grains; and to a lesser extent in green beans, sweet potatoes, potatoes, carrots, broccoli and berries.

I would like to thank Dr. Matt Dahlquist, DVM for correcting the text of this chapter and for offering many valuable suggestions and considerable help in its preparation.

8

Breeding

Captive-bred softbills have become more commonly available following advances in both avian nutrition and husbandry techniques; it is now quite easy to obtain aviary-bred shamas, blue-gray tanagers and even hummingbirds. There remains, however, the majority of softbills which are often not difficult to maintain, but still present a challenge to the aviculturist wishing to breed them.

Preferences of breeding pairs can vary tremendously, even if all are of the same species. It is therefore difficult to produce a blueprint for breeding softbills, but there are many techniques one can use to maximize the chances of success; and they are discussed in this chapter.

Sexing

Differences between the sexes of some softbills are clear and, provided they are mature, selecting a pair of such sexually dimorphic birds is easy. But many softbills are sexually monomorphic—the sexes are alike—making the visual selection of a pair impossible. Guesswork and intuition used to be relied upon, but nowadays a bird can be accurately and cheaply sexed using the following methods.

Surgical sexing

This is the most popular technique. It must be carried out by a veterinarian and, in expert hands, birds as small as a Pekin robin, *Leiothrix lutea*, can be safely sexed. A general anesthetic is normally used, and the procedure involves making a small incision in the abdominal wall through which a laparoscope is passed; the bird's gonads can then be inspected to determine the sex. The surgery does not usually require a suture and the post-operative care is often limited to a broad-spectrum antibiotic.

Not every veterinarian provides this service, but it is familiar to many, being appreciated also as a means of diagnosing ailments usually only revealed during an autopsy.

Chromosomal karyotyping

This method of sexing involves the laboratory analysis of the feather pulp from a young growing feather (a blood feather). The feather is analyzed for the presence of the sex chromosomes, known as ZY in the female and ZZ in the male; the two male chromosomes are the same length while one of the female's is much shorter than the other.

Birds' chromosomes tend to be more fragile than mammals', and the feather must be sent to the laboratory on an ice pack by overnight mail. In the United States, feather-pulp sexing can be done by Avian Genetic Sexing Laboratory, Barlette, TN.

DNA sexing

DNA sexing is another laboratory technique and involves analyzing the red blood cells to determine the presence of male or female chromosomes. Only one drop of blood is required and a veterinarian can obtain a sample; or a competent aviculturist can clip one of the bird's claws and drip blood into a container—a free collecting kit is usually provided for this purpose. The sample is then sent by regular mail to the laboratory.

Birds of any age can be sexed using this method and the blood sample has a relatively long shelf life without refrigeration. DNA fingerprinting to positively identify a bird's parentage is also available. In the United States, DNA sexing can be done by Zoogen Inc., Davis, CA.

Fecal steroid analysis

This involves testing a bird's droppings for the presence of reproductive hormones. It relies on measuring the relative levels of estrogen and testosterone of males and females of the same species. The baseline levels depend on the species and sex determination is unreliable. The bird must also be sexually mature for this method to work. In the United States, this sexing technique is offered by A.U.D. Laboratory, Aztec, NM.

Breeding Environment

Softbills can be nervous birds and become even more so during breeding. A secluded, well-planted and quiet aviary is therefore recommended. And if possible, air conditioning and heating units should be muffled to reduce their noise, since this may interfere with important courtship vocalizations. If the aviary can be approached from the side it should be screened. Feeding can be done through a hatch and cleaning in the main body of the enclosure should be greatly reduced or stopped during the breeding season.

Plant-life provides natural nest sites and seclusion, and attracts insects used by the vast majority of softbills to rear their young. Planted hanging baskets are of particular value often serving as nesting platforms. The nest is usually constructed in a depression scraped out by the softbills, although sometimes eggs are laid directly onto the soil. Camouflaged by the baskets' foliage such nests are very difficult to see, and watering the plants must be done with care.

Mixed species—pros and cons

Several species may live together amicably for much of the year; but if they are in peak condition, conflict can occur during the breeding season. If a pair does decide to breed they can be expected to chase intruders from the nest site, occasionally with fatal consequences. Equally other, more dominant, birds may injure the breeding pair or ransack their nest for eggs or useful nesting materials. Troupials, starlings and magpies are famous for this type of behavior, often making a nuisance of themselves as they poke about in other birds' nests.

With the hatching of chicks, a variety of live food will be needed. But in a mixed aviary, birds intent on feeding their young will have to compete with others for the choicest foods. Therefore, generally such an environment does not provide the ideal breeding conditions, and results are frequently best if a pair is housed alone. However, a very few softbills, such as bee eaters and white eyes, can live and breed in groups. Other species such as some jays, tanagers and hornbills may live as family groups with the juveniles helping to raise subsequent young.

Compatibility

Obtaining compatible pairs is often easiest if several specimens are purchased. If a long-term breeding program is undertaken, purchasing at least 20 percent extra birds is recommended, since by the time new blood is needed or losses occur, the species may not be so readily available. The softbills should be temporarily housed as a group; observations are then used to identify pairs which can be removed to separate breeding aviaries.

A pair of softbills will often live amicably together year-round. But sometimes the male reaches breeding condition before the female, and his unwanted advances can lead to fighting. The worst fighting usually occurs with solitary birds such as certain insectivores and toucans. It may be necessary to keep them apart. Ideally they should be in adjacent aviaries in visual contact. Hopefully, courtship displays and vocalizations will indicate readiness to breed, and an introduction can then be attempted. If the aviaries are interconnecting or separated by a sliding partition, the introduction can be stress-free. But fighting can still ensue and several attempts at pairing may have to be made. If all else fails, lightly clipping one of the aggressor's wings can give the weaker bird a helpful advantage.

If the birds cannot be housed in adjacent aviaries, one bird can be kept for a few days in a release ("howdie") cage within the main enclosure. Provided there is no aggression shown by either softbill, the howdied specimen can then be released.

Breeding Stimuli

The photoperiod

Provided with the correct nutrition and stimulated by an increasing photoperiod, birds can be encouraged to breed not only in the spring but also in the winter, when the hours of natural daylight are much shorter.

Lights can be operated by a dimmer switch: on a low setting

they can be used as a night light; set on full, they serve to extend the photoperiod. A light cycle of between 12 and 16 hours is often required for breeding, depending on the latitudes of the natural habitat—the higher the latitude, the longer the daylight hours must be to stimulate breeding.

A simple timer and dimmer switch can be used to give full lighting control. Advanced lighting systems can automatically reduce or increase light intensities to simulate dusk or dawn. Systems can even be adapted to illuminate the bird room if the natural light intensity falls below a preset level.

Rain

In the tropics, summer showers can be heavy but are usually short, and end as suddenly as they begin. The atmosphere becomes cooler and more humid until the sunshine emerges and life returns to normal.

These are ideal conditions for plant life. Nectar-filled blooms and fruits abound—all good foods in themselves, but more importantly they harbor a host of insects which are vital for the rearing of most softbills. Thus, in tropical regions it is the return of the rains and the passing of the dry season that can act as a breeding trigger for softbilled birds.

Artificial rain is easily produced by using a sprinkler system. The materials are very cheap and can be purchased from most garden centers. A length of tubing should be run along the top of the aviary and connected to a water tap. At regular intervals sprinkler heads can be fitted and these will emit an even distribution of "rain." The rain need only be turned on for ten minutes each day and care must be taken not to saturate food bowls or nesting sites.

The rain will bring a welcome relief from high summer temperatures and will encourage reluctant bathers to clean their plumage. It should not be used in the presence of fledglings or at temperatures much below 70°F (21.2°C) since some softbills will persist in bathing and may catch a chill.

Live food

In the wild, an increase of insects may trigger breeding activity, so in the aviary an abundance of live food can have a similar effect.

Spring is the time of plenty and combined with lengthening daylight hours, raising the live food content of a diet by about 30 percent can stimulate a potential breeding pair.

Temperature

Some parrot breeders raise the ambient temperature during the breeding season, with apparently enhanced results. For species that come from equatorial regions (and do not experience seasonal changes in day length), this may be an important breeding stimulus. However, better empirical data is still required, and in practice the best breeding stimuli are an increasing light cycle and more live food; and to a slightly lesser extent, the coming of the rains.

Nesting Receptacles

Many softbills prefer to build their nests in mature vegetation or a secluded cavity. But if the natural opportunities are not to their liking, artificial sites will very often be accepted.

Location

An assortment of nesting receptacles should be offered, fixed at different heights and in various locations, with one or two in the shelter. They are best located far from where people may stand and preferably in a well-planted spot—a small conifer branch fixed in front of the nest site can increase the feeling of seclusion. And remember that many nests are lost to heavy rain, so position receptacles beneath the flight's roofed sections.

Substrate

It is usually a good idea to add about 4 in. (10 cm) of wood shavings to the nest box—do not use sawdust as this can cause various respiratory and eye problems. Most softbills will then kick out enough shavings to suit their needs and build a nest on the remaining base. If all of the shavings are persistently kicked from the box, and breeding activity does not occur, it can be helpful to introduce a heavier medium such as soil or a square of turf. Equally, a deeper nesting box may be needed, especially in the case of very large softbills. Birds with powerful, destructive bills such as toucans, hornbills and barbets are often happiest making their own substrate.

Strips of soft or rotting wood can be left in the box for the softbills to chew up themselves.

Hygiene

The interior of a nest box can get very hot and humid in the summer and may encourage the growth of fungi. To reduce the risk of diseases such as aspergillosis, ventilation within the box should be promoted. Small holes can be drilled along the top, on opposing sides, or the lid prevented from fully closing. At the end of each breeding season, thoroughly clean and disinfect the boxes and leave them out to dry in direct sunlight.

Platforms

Fruit pigeons and doves are not usually gifted architects, and if they can be persuaded to use an artificial site, success will be more likely. A square platform made of wire mesh or wood is suitable, and some birds prefer the greater depth of an empty hanging basket. All should be lined with materials such as coconut fibers and twigs, to both encourage breeding and protect the eggs. The softbills may then bring their own materials to the nest and complete the characteristic mishmash of twigs. Touracos tend to build equally flimsy platform-type nests and should be offered the same receptacles. Members of the crow family also accept such receptacles and typically build a strong nest of twigs.

Cup-shaped nests

A number of species make use of cup-shaped wicker or metal receptacles marketed for canaries. The smaller babblers such as Pekin robins, mesias, minlas and fulvettas may nest in them along with certain flycatchers, yuhinas, white eyes, bearded reedlings and tanagers.

Laughing thrushes, sibias, fairy bluebirds and *Chloropsis* tend to prefer slightly larger sites such as empty or planted hanging baskets and occasionally the nest of a wild thrush may be accepted. The nests of American robins, *Turdus migratorius*, are ideal and at the very least provide good materials for the softbills to construct their own nests—wild birds' nests must be thoroughly cleaned and disinfected before use, since they can be infested with red mites. (See also Ailments—mites and lice.)

Half-open-fronted boxes

All of the species that build cup-shaped nests should be provided with a half-open-fronted box. I have seen flycatchers, niltavas, *Chloropsis*, shamas, tanagers, mesias, Pekin robins and Mount Omei liocichlas use such an offering where other receptacles were ignored. Variations on the basic design are recommended with an almost fully open front suitable for softbills of fairy bluebird size.

Parakeet-type boxes

Species that nest in tree holes will often accept a parakeet-type box of a horizontal or, the more familiar, upright design. Mynahs and starlings will rarely refuse such a box. Large versions of the upright design are suitable for barbets and woodpeckers; and boxes as tall as 5 ft. (1.5 m) may be needed for the bigger hornbill and toucan species—a hollowed-out palm log is even better. In miniature, the same design will suit most tits and nuthatches. Occasionally shamas, redstarts and flycatchers will use a parakeet box, although a half-open-fronted design is usually their preference.

Nesting Materials

Some birds merely visit nest boxes to satisfy their inquisitive nature or to roost. But if material is repeatedly carried to a specific location, nest building is probably underway.

Paper and cobwebs

Thin, dried twigs, dried grasses, animal hair, wool, rootlets, mosses and strips of paper are all ideal nest-building materials. And for the nest lining, the down from a plant, small feathers and even washing/drying machine lint can be offered. Vital for hummingbirds and sunbirds are cobwebs: the silk is wrapped around the nest and used as a kind of adhesive. Without the silk, nests could still be built, but would be prone to collapse.

Mud

This is important in the breeding of some softbills, most famous of which is the hornbill. The female of nearly all hornbill species is sealed into the nesting chamber behind a wall of feces and sticky foods, with many species also using mud.

Nuthatches can also use mud for nesting as they modify the

entrance hole with a mud-clay plaster. The work is sometimes considerable and protects the nest by reducing the entrance to the smallest possible aperture. The western rock nuthatch, *Sitta neumayer*, takes this technique one step further by using mud to build an entire flask-shaped nest, which it lodges in rock work.

Many members of the crow family, such as magpies and jays, will use mud to bind their nests of twigs together during the initial stages of construction. Mud is also used by some thrushes to reinforce their nests or glue them to a suitable base. And the now considerable avicultural rarities, the cocks-of-the-rock, build nests of mud and saliva while the even rarer horneros make a domed, oven-like structure.

Rearing

Many softbills are extremely surreptitious in their nest building, and in a well-planted aviary the smaller species are quite capable of building a nest and even incubating its eggs without your knowledge. Good observations are therefore essential in order to properly cater to the needs of the new family. Equally, if the eggs fail to hatch they can be promptly removed, allowing the pair to recycle and lay a fresh clutch. If at all possible, observations should be done without entering the breeding aviary. Although a nest is unlikely to be deserted if disturbed, it may be left long enough for the eggs to become chilled.

Incubation

Some softbills such as cuckoos, hornbills, bee eaters, kingfishers, hummingbirds and touracos begin incubation with the laying of the first egg; the chicks therefore hatch asynchronously a day or so apart. However, the majority of softbills begin incubation once the clutch is complete or nearly complete. As a consequence the eggs hatch at approximately the same time and, hatching synchronously or semi-synchronously, the chicks are more or less the same size. So as not to attract predators the neatly severed egg shells are normally dropped as far from the nest as possible. But in the confines of an aviary the shells are often obvious and provide the first real evidence of a successful hatch. However, birds such as touracos and members of the crow family usually consume the shells.

Rearing foods

The vast majority of softbills become highly insectivorous when rearing young—omnivores feed their chicks almost exclusively on insects for the first week or so. It is the urgency for live food that can betray a nest, since birds often reluctant to show themselves become far bolder in their search for insects. If you suspect the presence of young, it is frequently revealing to place extra live food in the aviary and watch the birds' reactions. Hopefully one or both adults will take live food and, without eating it themselves, fly to the nest. If this action is repeated, the existence of chicks can be inferred, and it is probably unnecessary to inspect the nest and risk disturbing the birds.

Live food

Mealworms, waxworms and crickets represent good rearing food for most softbills—they should be offered in plenty and regularly replenished. It is important to sprinkle a multivitamin and mineral supplement on the rearing food to prevent rickets. (See also Ailments—rickets.)

Smaller birds and especially insectivores will sometimes show a preference for feeding ant pupae to their young. This highly nutritious food cannot be purchased, but should be collected in the summer months and used immediately; or it can be frozen and kept for future use. Fruit flies are valuable for tiny insectivores and nectivores, as well as aphids which can be attracted to the aviary by planting rose bushes in the flight. Maggots can be allowed to metamorphose into flies, to provide an absolutely indispensable rearing food for flycatchers.

Chick eating and carnivores

The more carnivorous softbills such as toucans, hornbills, shrikes, kingfishers and certain barbets often need chopped or whole pinkie mice when rearing chicks. A very plentiful supply of such foods should be furnished since the quest for live food is so intense, the parents may otherwise eat their own young. This unfortunate practice can become a vice, much like egg-eating, and can be exceptionally difficult to cure.

Conversely, certain individuals seem more prone to eating or injuring their young, precisely when too much live food is supplied. With their need to search for food removed, the adults appear to get bored and turn on their family. Most of the more carnivorous softbills are susceptible to this "boredom syndrome" and can benefit from a short search for food. Techniques I have used for jays, magpies and shrikes include burying foods in a tray of bran, hiding foods about the aviary and offering small amounts of food at regular intervals. Such ploys extend the searching time and occupy these often very intelligent birds.

Fruit doves and pigeons

Unlike the majority of softbills, fruit pigeons and doves have no need for live food during the rearing process, and do not need any special foods. This is because they have evolved the ability to produce "crop milk," a creamy secretion that totally nourishes the chick for the first few days. Thereafter, it receives a mixture of milk and the adult food.

Breeding Problems

Chicks fallen from the nest

This can happen either as a result of their own exuberance or as they are accidentally caught by the foot of a departing parent. Often a dead body is discovered on the aviary floor—usually early in the morning—but if life persists, the chick should be held in cupped hands and warm air gently breathed onto it. Occasionally, even apparently dead birds will be revived in this way and they can then be returned to the nest; to distract the adults and lessen the commotion a fresh dish of live food should be provided. If the chick is not accepted, hand rearing may have to be considered, especially if there has been a history of parental failure. (See also Hand Rearing on page 97.)

Egg eating

Adults sometimes develop a taste for their own eggs and repeatedly eat them. I have never had any success with old-fashioned remedies such as filling dummy eggs with hot foods like Tabasco sauce. In practice, the best course of action is to take the eggs for artificial incubation. The chick can then be hand reared; or quite often the adults will accept the newly hatched chick, provided they had previously been incubating a dummy egg. Simply encourage the incubating bird from the nest, remove the dummy egg and replace it with the newly hatched chick (with shell halves still around it). If an adult returns to the nest and resumes normal brooding, then all is likely to be well.

Parental chick plucking

Like egg eating, this is another vice which is very difficult, if not impossible, to cure. But the course of action is straight forward: once the chick has reached fledging age, put it in a cage and the parents will continue to feed it through the wire mesh. Place the cage in the shelter at about 70°F (21.1°C) to prevent the plucked youngster from catching a chill. The chick will be protected from plucking, and normal plumage should return with the next molt. However, if the follicles have been damaged by the parents' plucking (which tends to be seen more in parrots), the return of normal plumage is far less certain.

Dangers of fledging

Caging chicks at fledging time is also a very good way of protecting them from the dangers of fledging. The young continue to be fed by their parents through the wire mesh while being protected in the cage—many chicks otherwise perish in planted enclosures as they disappear in the undergrowth or are attacked by other birds. Alternatively, the young can be taken from the aviary and fed by hand.

9

Rings, Records and Studbooks

Leg Bands

It is often necessary to identify a bird with a unique number which relates to a studbook or ancestral chart. Leg bands are a good way of achieving this and there are 2 types of bands available.

Closed bands

Closed or "seamless" bands are used to denote a captive-bred bird, since they can only be fitted when the bird is only a few days old. At this age the toes are small and the bones of the foot are soft, allowing the hind toe to be bent back parallel to the leg, and the ring can be slid over the foot. The foot quickly grows and the bones harden to make such a ring a permanent sign of captive breeding.

Occasionally young chicks have been taken from the wild, banded and imported as captive-bred ones. Fortunately such practices seem to be rare, and can be uncovered by using DNA fingerprinting techniques to determine a bird's true parentage.

Closed bands are most often used on hand-reared birds. But if parent-reared birds (that remain in the nest) are to be banded, you must be very careful, because some parents will throw the chick from the nest in an effort to remove the foreign object. Make the bands less conspicuous by darkening them with a black pen, and wait until the evening when the adults are less active. Also, try to band the chicks when they are 8 to 10 days old, so that if they are rejected, they will be easier to hand rear.

It may be a legal requirement to closed band the softbills you breed, depending on state or federal laws, the species and whether the birds are to be sold or exhibited. Check with the U.S. Fish &

Wildlife Service, bird clubs or zoos in your area (or the Department of the Environment in U.K.).

Open bands

Available in plastic or metal, they have a joint in them so they can be fitted on an adult bird's leg. The metal bands are fitted with a tool, similar to a pair of pliers, which closes the band onto the leg. This is a delicate and potentially dangerous procedure, because birds' legs are fragile and very easily broken. If you feel nervous, ask for help. Banding is always much easier and safer with 2 people.

It is important to use a band of the correct size to avoid injury. Bands that are too tight can cause gangrene and the loss of the entire foot. Equally if the band is too loose, it can slip down over the foot resulting in similar damage.

In the United States, all legally imported birds pass through federal quarantine where they are fitted with an open metal band that bears the unique marks of the quarantine station.

Colored bands

Colored bands are very good for identifying birds at a distance. Open bands are available in several colors and they also have a unique number on them. But if you just want a color ID, a small, colored cable tie will identify a bird as Pink-Left (leg) for example.

Records

It is extremely beneficial to keep a file on each bird describing the complete life history: future breeding programs can be fine tuned and medical problems more easily assessed. If you have a computer, a print out of a bird's history is very useful for a new owner, and will reflect well on your general approach to animal management. Since most birds are regulated in some way by law, a well-presented and thorough record of each bird's history can be invaluable. This type of record will also be especially helpful if you wish to participate in any kind of formal breeding program or studbook.

Example record for adult specimen
- Report date: May 16 1996
- Latin name: *Niltava grandis* Acquired: 16 May 1995
- Common name: Greater Niltava ID: 1423 Pink Right

- Age: 3 years Sex: Female
- Aviary: No. 4
- Captive hatch: 3 May 1993 (hand reared)
- Dam: 1648 owned by Mr. X
- Sire: 9915 owned by Mr. X
- Purchased from Mr. X $90.
- Breeding rating out of 10: 9

    History

- Breeding: 18 July 1995
- Incubating in half-open-fronted box
- Breeding: 2 August 1995
- Taking waxworms to box
- Breeding: 18 August 1995
- 2 chicks fledge, 1 dead in box
- Medical: 5 December 1995
- Tangled nest fibers removed from foot by vet, and band removed to help recovery.

Studbooks

Studbooks have been in existence for more than 150 years and were originally developed to regulate poultry and livestock. They still protect the pedigrees of many of our domesticated animals, but serve another vital function as a zoological tool for the preservation of threatened and endangered species. A studbook is fundamental to the success of any long-term breeding program, as it details the complete history of the captive population including births, deaths, sex and family lineage. With computer analysis, genetics and demographics, a modern studbook can develop a self-sustaining (genetically diverse) captive population. This is especially important if any of the studbook animals are introduced back into the wild; the fact that the population is unrelated, and more able to adapt to change, helps to ensure their long-term survival.

Zoos tend to operate studbooks, under the auspices of the AZA (American Zoo and Aquarium Association). But private aviculturists are often included, and in terms of expertise, aviary space and good quality birds, bring much to the conservation effort.

AZA approved softbill studbooks

At present there are twenty-two studbooks for softbill species. If you would like more information on them, your local zoo will be glad to help; or you can contact the American Zoo and Aquarium Association at: Executive Office and Conservation Center, 7970-D Old Georgetown Road, Bethesda, MD, 20814-2493; (301) 907-7777 Fax: 907-2980.

Fairy bluebird, *Irena puella*
Dove, Black-naped fruit, *Ptilinopus melanospila*
Dove, Jambu fruit, *Ptilinopus jambu*
Dove, Marianas fruit, *Ptilinopus roseicapillus*
Dove, Temminck's fruit, *Ptilinopus porphyrea*
Frogmouth, Tawney, *Podargus strigoides*
Hornbill, Abyssinian ground, *Bucorvus abyssinicus*
Hornbill, Great, *Buceros bicornis*
Hornbill, Rhinoceros, *Buceros rhinoceros*
Hornbill, Rufous, *Buceros hydrocorax*
Kingfisher, Giant, *Megaceryle torquata*
Kingfisher, Guam, *Halcyon cinnamomina cinnamomina*
Kookaburra, Laughing, *Dacelo novaeguineae*
Mynah, Bali, *Leucopsar rothschildi*
Rail, Guam, *Rallus owstoni*
Roller, Lilac-breasted, *Coracias caudata*
Sunbittern, *Eurypyga helias*
Tanager, Blue-gray, *Thraupis episcopus*
Tanager, Silver-beaked, *Ramphocelus carbo*
Tanager, Turquoise, *Tangara mexicana*
Toucan, Toco, *Ramphastos toco*
Touraco, Violet, *Musophaga violacea*

10

Incubation and Hand Rearing

Artificial incubation and hand rearing have evolved to become a reliable and practical tool in the breeding of softbills. And even previously unrearable birds, such as fruit doves and pigeons, can now be hand reared from the egg.

Incubation

Egg cleaning

When a freshly laid egg cools, it sucks in some of the atmosphere around it. Since it is often impractical to keep nest sites scrupulously clean, this represents a hazard to the developing embryo, as potentially lethal bacteria can be absorbed. The egg should therefore be cleaned with a suitable egg disinfectant, such as diluted Nolvasan™, safeguarding not only the individual egg but the entire contents of your incubator.

The sterilizing liquid should be warmer than the incubated egg at 110°–120°F (43°–49°C): this causes the bacteria in the shell's pores to be pushed out and destroyed as they mix with the solution. Dip the egg briefly in the liquid, and hold it carefully since it will now be very slippery. If you are cleaning a cold egg that has not yet been incubated, allow it to warm up to room temperature for at least 30 minutes before dipping it.

Handling

Once cleaned, the egg must be handled with thoroughly scrubbed hands, and very preferably latex gloves should be worn: even the oil on your hands can affect the protective outer surface of the egg, called the cuticle or bloom. Generally the egg should not be subjected to any sudden movements or jolts. Care should also be taken not to point the blunt end of the egg downwards since this may strain the membranes between the albumen and airspace. Holding the egg on its side is preferable.

Storing

This is usually only done with precocial birds such as pheasants and waterfowl and is not normally necessary for softbills. The very small eggs of most softbill species do not store particularly well and should be incubated as soon as possible after collection—the fresher the egg the more likely it is to hatch.

The Incubator

Hygiene

The conditions inside an incubator are ideal for the growth of bacteria. It is therefore important to clean the machine every few weeks and especially at the beginning of the breeding season.

Many incubators come apart completely to facilitate thorough cleaning. The components can then be scrubbed, preferably while submerged in a bath of disinfectant. Once dried and reassembled, the cleaning process may be completed by gassing the incubator using formaldehyde crystals. The crystals can be purchased from gardening suppliers, and are put onto a dish inside the incubator, heated and allowed to become gaseous. The machine is then turned on, to propel the gas into every nook and cranny.

Caution: exposure to the gas may be harmful to people and especially animals. Work away from your birds in a well-ventilated room or outside.

Temperature

In the wild, birds sometimes leave their eggs unattended for many minutes while defending the nest or feeding. This, and changes in the eggs' positions within the nest, help vary the incubation temperature which facilitates calcium metabolism from the shell to the embryo. An occasional, brief cooling of the eggs may therefore be beneficial; and this is usually achieved when the incubator door is opened for routine egg inspection.

A stable, average temperature is essential, however; and softbill eggs are often incubated at a dry-bulb temperature of about 99.5°F (37.5°C) and a wet-bulb temperature of approximately 84°F (28.9°C) and RH 53%. But these figures are based on the egg of a domestic chicken, which has an incubation period of twenty-one days. Softbill eggs are often of a different size and/or have a different incubation period. For them, 99.5°F is not necessarily the ideal dry-bulb temperature, and account should be taken of the egg's size before incubation begins.

Small eggs: research indicates that eggs smaller than domestic chicken eggs, with an incubation period less than twenty-one days, generally require a dry-bulb temperature equal to, or greater than, 99.5°F (37.5°C). Eggs of the following softbills tend to do best at 100.6°F (38.1°C) with a wet bulb temperature of 86°–88°F (30°–31.1°C) and RH 58%: Crows, barbets, fairy bluebird, fruit doves, jays, kingfishers, laughing thrushes, magpies, mynahs, Pekin robin, shrikes, silver-eared mesia, starlings, tanagers, thrushes, woodpeckers and yuhinas.

Large eggs: eggs larger than domestic chicken eggs with an incubation period greater than twenty-one days, usually need a dry-bulb temperature lower than 99.5°F (37.5°C). Eggs of the following softbills tend to do best at 99°F (37.2°C) with a wet-bulb temperature of 86°–88°F (30°–31.1°C) and RH 64.5%: Aracaris, avocets, cocks of the rock, gallinules, kookaburras, plovers, rails, sunbittern, tawney frogmouth, toucans and touracos.

Very large eggs: the larger the egg, the more the incubation temperature needs to be below 99.5°F (37.5°C). For example, the egg of the brown kiwi, *Apteryx australis mantelli*, does best at 97.5°F (36.4°C) with a wet-bulb temperature of 82°–84.9°F (27.8°–29.4°C). (Kuehler and Good 1990.)

You will know if the incubation temperature is correct for a given species by comparing the period of artificial incubation with the natural (parental) incubation period. They should be the same or very similar to help ensure a healthy chick. If the egg takes too long to hatch, the incubation temperature may be too low, while an early hatch may be caused by a high temperature.

Thermometers

Accurately measuring the temperature of your incubator is vital for success. Eggs can still hatch when incubated at the wrong temperature but may produce weak or deformed chicks; and often an incorrect incubation temperature will cause early death of the embryo.

Thermometers can vary considerably in their accuracy and it is a good idea to compare a new thermometer with that of a friend who is successful at incubation. A local zoo, hospital or laboratory will usually be glad to test a thermometer for you. Digital thermometers are easier to read although no more reliable than mercury devices.

In a still-air incubator there is a significant heat gradient, with the top of the incubator being much hotter than the bottom. The position of the thermometer is therefore important, and it should be placed at the same level as the eggs. In a moving (forced) air incubator, position of the thermometer is not as crucial since there is a fairly even temperature distribution throughout the machine.

Humidity

Measuring and controlling humidity is important, and vital if weight-loss techniques are to be used. Some incubators have automatic humidity controls, and for those that do not, kits can be purchased to make the necessary conversion.

But the majority of incubators rely on wet-bulb thermometers for the measurement of humidity. These are ordinary mercury thermometers connected to a wick; the wick is kept wet by being permanently dipped in water, and as the water evaporates over the thermometer it indicates the level of humidity. If the air is dry it will draw water from the wick and cool the thermometer, leading to a low humidity reading; and vice versa.

The humidity necessary for correct incubation can be supplied by allowing dishes of distilled water to evaporate within the machine. To prevent these dishes from acting as reservoirs for bacteria they should contain a suitable incubator disinfectant such as Nolvasan™ or EnviroClean™.

Experience will quickly determine the best wet-bulb reading for a particular species. A good point to start at is 84°F (28.9°C) with a dry-bulb reading of 99.5°F (37.5°C) and RH 53%.

Testing

To be on the safe side, it is best to have an incubator running for a few weeks before it is needed. This will give enough time to fully test it and ensure that everything is functioning consistently. The temperature and humidity must be regularly checked and recorded. Then, if necessary, the incubator can be adjusted at the end of the day. Readings will vary somewhat throughout the day and waiting until later in the day is the best way of achieving accurate results.

The entire setup can go through a dress rehearsal by incubating a number of chicken eggs. This will be an important confidence booster, and if there is a disaster the loss will not be too great.

The Incubation Process

Weight loss

During incubation an egg steadily loses weight as the fat from the yolk is metabolized to provide energy for the growing embryo. Weight is also lost as moisture leaves the egg along with gaseous metabolic waste from the embryo.

Charting the weight loss: preferably done on a daily basis, this can significantly increase hatch rates as the egg's progress is accurately monitored. By the time the egg is due to hatch, it should have lost approximately 12 to 15 percent (see chart) of its freshly laid weight. If the shell's thickness is normal, and the temperature and humidity are correct, this happens naturally and the chick hatches without incident. Sometimes an egg will lose weight too quickly or too slowly, and prompt corrective action is required to insure a normal hatch.

Example weight loss chart

Egg weighs 8 grams when laid.
Incubation period is 14 days.
Point a = 8
Point b = 8 - (8 x 0.12) = 7.04
Point c = 8 - (8 x 0.15) = 6.8

Plot the egg's weight each day. To ensure a healthy hatch, the plotted points should remain within the boundaries. If they stray, control the weight loss by altering the level of humidity in the incubator.

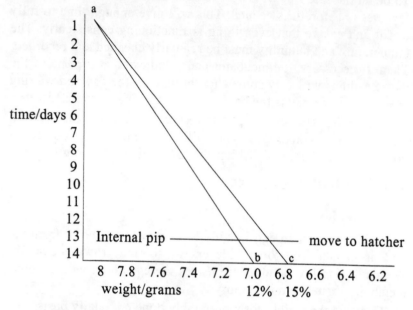

Controlling the rate of weight loss: this is done by altering the level of humidity in the incubator. If the egg is losing too much weight the level of humidity must be increased; and vice versa. Because changing the humidity will affect every egg in the incubator, it is best to operate two or three small incubators, each with slightly different humidity levels—a difference of about 10°F on the wet-bulb thermometer is usually sufficient. Individual eggs can then be moved to the most appropriate humidity, and if necessary can be moved repeatedly to maintain the correct weight loss.

The correct level of humidity must be arrived at before the egg has completed 30 percent of its incubation, because the rate of weight loss is very difficult to change after this point. It is therefore desirable to let the parents incubate the egg for the first 30 percent of the incubation period to set the correct weight loss pattern.

Very thin or thick-shelled eggs: for some eggs, simply altering the level of humidity cannot adequately control their weight loss. Very thin-shelled eggs will lose weight extremely fast while especially thick-shelled ones will refuse to lose hardly any weight at all. Fortunately such eggs are rare, but if they are to hatch, drastic action must be taken.

Unusually thin-shelled eggs can be coated in nail polish or covered with cling wrap to reduce the porosity of the shell, thus slowing the rate of weight loss. Using cling wrap is preferable because it can be reduced or periodically removed to allow the normal gas exchange of the egg: as the embryo develops, it exchanges carbon dioxide for oxygen through the pores of the shell. But the embryo can die if this exchange is impaired, especially in the latter stages of incubation when the gas exchange is at its greatest.

In the case of thick-shelled eggs, a tiny hole can be delicately made into the air space, allowing moisture to escape and hence weight to be lost. Equally, the shell can be made more porous by gently sanding it; or the cuticle can be bleached away by dipping the egg in a 10 percent bleach solution at 110°–120°F (43°–49°C) (Fox 1995).

Repairing damaged eggs

Provided the shell membranes are unbroken and lethal bacteria has not entered the egg, cracks and minor shell damage can be successfully repaired with various substances such as nail polish, typewriter correction fluid, Vetbond™ or superglue. But be aware that the repairing fluid will reduce the porosity of the shell, and if the affected area is large enough, the egg's weight loss characteristics could be significantly altered.

Candling

Shining a bright light into most eggs reveals their stage of development and even a beating heart can be seen in the more mature embryo. Candling is started at the blunt end of the egg but once the embryo is more developed, viewing from the pointed end is better. By the time 60 percent of the incubation is complete, the entire egg should be covered with veins. From this point onward, changes in growth are not usually appreciable.

Turning

Automatic turning is very popular and prevents the operator from forgetting to turn the eggs. Eggs can be stood upright in a tray and tilted from side to side; or they can be laid horizontally and rotated by means of rollers or a moving "carpet."

Many eggs develop and hatch successfully in an upright position. But softbill eggs tend to do much better when incubated in a horizontal position, and turned a full 180° at least every hour. Turning should be alternated between clockwise and counterclockwise to prevent twisting of the chalazae—cords of protein (albumin) that suspend the yolk in the center of the egg. With automatic turners that continuously turn in the same direction, the chalazae can be protected by manually rotating the egg 180° along its horizontal axis, twice a day.

Turning versus yolk size

The yolk in many softbill eggs represents less than about 30 percent of the total egg mass. This compares with larger yolks of at least 35 percent in most pheasants and at least 40 percent in most waterfowl.

Larger-yolked eggs can be successfully hatched using any conventional method of turning. But for the small-yolked eggs of many softbills, high turning rates (from 30 to 60 times a day) can lead to considerably improved hatching results. As well as the rate of turning, it is equally important to incubate the egg horizontally, rather than vertically. (Harvey 1993.)

Hatching

The chick is very vulnerable once it begins to hatch. When the shell is broken, the membranes can quickly dry out if the air around them is not extremely humid. The chick can become sticky and unable to rotate within the egg; and as the membranes become tough and rubbery, the chick will need to be helped from the egg or risk dying.

To avoid such problems the egg should be transferred to a separate hatching incubator, once the chick has internally pipped (entered the airspace). At this point, the egg no longer needs to be turned and doing so will hinder the hatching process. Internal pipping may occur a day or so before hatching, although the exact time is variable and must be monitored by candling. The chick is now breathing air from the airspace, and is fully formed and about to begin hatching (external pipping).

The hatching incubator should be at maximum humidity and can be a moving or still-air design. Generally, small softbill eggs should be hatched at the same dry-bulb temperature used for their incubation. However, the larger eggs tend to hatch better at about 1°F lower than the incubation temperature, since warmth is generated during the hatch and the eggs may otherwise overheat.

Parent birds often stimulate hatching by communicating with the chick while it's still in the egg. In an incubator, hatching may be encouraged by playing recorded vocalizations of the adults.

Hand Rearing

With a little practice, hand rearing can be an invaluable breeding aid, especially when combined with artificial incubation. Some birds develop a history of failure, and softbills that would otherwise break, eat or poorly incubate their eggs, or fail to raise their young, can benefit from human intervention.

Equally, birds that are good parents can be made more productive by multiple clutching. This occurs when a clutch is taken for artificial incubation and rearing, in the hope that a replacement clutch will be laid. Often this occurs within 2 or 3 weeks and can be left with the parents, given to foster parents or artificially incubated and hand reared. If the eggs are taken from the parents, yet another clutch can be expected and in this way the productivity of just one pair of softbills can be amazing.

Hygiene

Wash your hands thoroughly before doing any work in the hand-rearing area.

Ensure that the feeding utensils are properly cleaned and disinfected in a solution such as Nolvasan™. Disinfectants are inactivated by organic matter, such as food remains, so clean the utensils thoroughly in water before disinfection. It is also important to soak the utensils for at least 15 minutes before they can be considered properly cleaned, since disinfectants do not work instantly. Replace the disinfectant solution at least every third day to maintain its effectiveness. Take time to thoroughly rinse utensils before use, since some products, like bleach, may be lethal if ingested. Syringes can become sticky after a period of soaking, so if necessary use a cooking oil spray to lubricate them and temporarily restore their smooth action.

Using only one syringe or pair of tweezers to feed several chicks is a means of disease transference. Try to avoid "double dipping" by providing a feeding implement for every chick.

Immediately after Hatching

The first 12 to 24 hours

Spray or swab the umbilicus with iodine solution; and leave the chick in the hatcher for several hours, where it can dry off and recover from the exertions of hatching. During this period it does not need to be fed and doing so can interfere with the normal absorption of the yolk sac. This in turn can make the chick more vulnerable to egg peritonitis, an infection caused by the escape of yolk material into the body cavity. An oral electrolyte, such as Pedialyte™, can be fed during the first 24 hours to prevent dehydration, but even this is often not necessary.

Temperature

The newly hatched chick will need to be kept in a brooder at 95°–99°F (35°–37.2°C) and at a humidity level similar to that used during incubation. The requirements of individual chicks can vary, but generally, if the bird is restless or panting it is probably too hot, while chicks that are lethargic or shivering may be cold.

As the softbill grows the temperature should gradually be reduced; otherwise the stress induced by overheating will be harmful, predisposing the youngster to develop such diseases as aspergillosis. Once the bird is fully feathered it will be comfortable at room temperature.

Floor covering

The chick should be placed in a margarine tub, or similar container, on a layer of very thin twigs, toweling or artificial fiber matting such as Enkamat™. Enkamat is an erosion-control matting made by Akzo Industrial Systems Company, P.O. Box 7249, Asheville, NC, 28802. Even newly hatched chicks can have quite strong feet and benefit from something to grip onto from day 1. This can help prevent irreversible leg and foot problems as the feet will grip and develop naturally. Wood shavings or hay can also be used, but be aware that species with particularly large gapes will try to swallow them, especially frogmouths, owlet-nightjars and the nightjars.

Growth is rapid and many passerine softbills leave the nest at only two weeks of age. At this point it is very important to provide suitable twigs and branches for the youngster to perch on, as it starts to explore its environment and while its feet are still developing.

Food

Recipes

Numerous foods can be used during the hand rearing of softbills; I prefer to use two different recipes. In both cases a probiotic preparation should be used according to the manufacturer's instructions. This preparation will help generate the gut flora necessary for normal digestion and will also provide important protection against pathogens such as *E. coli*.

Omnivore/frugivore

Do not feed for the first 24 hours. (See immediately after hatching.)

Day 1 to 6 approximately: 70 percent proprietary parrot rearing formula (I prefer Kaytee Exact™) premixed with water according to the manufacturer's instructions + 15 percent pureed apple + 15 percent pureed papaya. Blend together.

From day 6 approximately: thicken the food; and begin offering sliced pinkie mice and small pieces of the adult diet.

Insectivore/carnivore

Do not feed for the first 24 hours. (See immediately after hatching.)

Day 1 to 6 approximately: equal parts of whole raw egg, pinkie mice, waxworms, cricket abdomens and papaya. Mix in a food processor and add a multivitamin and mineral supplement.

Grind the ingredients into very small pieces if feeding with tweezers. If a syringe, eye dropper or spoon is used, puree the food and mix together to a liquidy-toothpaste consistency.

From day 6 approximately: thicken the food; and begin offering sliced pinkie mice and chopped insects. Dip the insects in water and sprinkle with a very fine insectivorous food.

Food temperature

The food must be between 100° and 106°F (37.8° and 41.1°C). A small thermometer will confirm the temperature and is more accurate and hygienic than tasting the food yourself. If the food is too cold the chick is likely to refuse it, while food that is too hot can result in crop burn. This injury can also be caused by food that is heated in a microwave oven, as hot spots can occur if the food is not thoroughly mixed. (See problems during hand rearing—crop burn.)

If only one syringe of food is required, it can be safely and quickly heated by holding it under running, hot water. During the feeding process, the food cools very quickly and can be kept warm by floating it in a pan of hot water.

Feeding

Feeding implements

Use a 1 cc syringe or eye dropper to start with, and as the chick grows, progress onto a larger syringe. You may prefer to use a spoon with its edges bent upward to mimic the parents' mandibles. While this method is slower and messier, it is safer because it does not force food into the chick's mouth which could cause it to aspirate (inhale) food. (See problems during hand rearing—aspiration.)

Instead of feeding a liquidy diet with a syringe or eye dropper, tweezers can be used to feed individual pieces of food from day one. This greatly reduces the risk of aspiration. But take care to feed extremely small food pieces that are easily digested, and ensure that the full range of foods are fed to deliver proper nutrition.

Feeding technique

Before feeding, it is important that you elicit a normal feeding response, otherwise food can more easily enter the trachea (windpipe) and be aspirated (inhaled). Whether using a spoon, syringe or tweezers, food should be delivered over the tongue, and the bird given an opportunity to swallow.

The esophagus runs down the right hand side of the neck (your left as you face the bird). Angling the syringe toward this side of the mouth might help prevent aspiration of food into the trachea, which passes down the center of the neck. But if the chick is willing, and the hand feeding is correct, it should not matter which side of the mouth the food enters.

How much to feed

It is essential that the chick is never overfed. Careful monitoring of the crop during feedings is a good way to ensure overfeeding doesn't occur. However, my preference is to deliver a measured amount of food from a syringe or weigh the chick before and after it has been fed. This is a more precise method of feeding and works equally well for those softbilled species that do not have a crop.

Overfeeding during the first week is a common error, and a common cause of death is aspiration of the liquidy diet. It is best to feed small amounts often, and as an example an aracari only needs about 0.2 cc per feeding for the first day. The interval between feeds (one to two hours for the first week) should allow the food to be easily digested; and the food should easily clear the crop for species that have one.

As a very rough guide, increase the amount fed each day by about 10 percent. But do not feed if there is still food in the crop from the previous feeding, as this can cause sour crop. (See problems during hand feeding—sour crop.)

After several days the chick will enter a phase of very fast growth. It is now extremely important not to underfeed, otherwise growth will be stunted, causing irreversible and eventually fatal retardation. A stunted chick is likely to have a grotesquely large head, with eyes still closed long after they should have opened.

Weight gain

A healthy chick should gain weight each day until the point of weaning. A zero weight gain, and particularly a loss in weight, is often the first sign of trouble. The bird may be underfed or sick; or the food may be too dilute or low in protein.

The bird's body should look in proportion and be a good weight for its size. The breast should be plump and rounded without a prominent keel. Equally the youngster must not be too fat since this can also be unhealthy, making liver and kidney disease more likely.

Day 1 to 6 approximately

It is important for the young chick to be well hydrated. A liquidy diet is therefore essential, as it is easily digested and absorbed. About 70 percent of the very first feed should be water or Pedialyte™. Feeds should be every hour or 2 between about 6 A.M. and midnight, and a 3 A.M. feed is highly recommended for the first 6 days.

From day 6 approximately

For softbills that normally fledge at about 14 days, larger feeds every 3 or 4 hours can now be given. But for species that fledge at about 21 days, the feeding frequency should not be reduced until the chick is approximately 11 days old.

A thicker, more nutritious food is necessary to fuel the fast growth that by now will be underway. See previous page. At this point the chick will be able to receive small pieces of the adult diet, plus slices of pinkie mice dipped in pureed fruits or vegetables—"stage one" human baby foods are highly nutritious and ideal for this purpose.

As the chick grows, the amount of adult food can be increased until the youngster is able to feed itself.

Weaning

Weaning, though not usually difficult, can be made even easier if a similar softbill is within view that can teach by example. A dish of the adult diet and a dish of water, should be left in the young bird's cage and eventually food will be played with and eaten. It is surprising how soon some birds start to feed themselves; and generally it is worth leaving food and water in the cage from about one to two weeks after the normal fledging time. Holding the dish of food up to the bird's face may encourage it to eat for itself. Hand feeding should still be used to supplement the bird's intake until it is fully independent.

Throughout the hand-rearing process, weighing the chick each day can provide an early warning of any problems. During the weaning period, a small, temporary decrease in weight is normal and is nature's way of encouraging the bird to feed itself.

Fruit Pigeons and Doves

Unlike other softbills, fruit pigeons and doves feed their young a highly nutritious crop milk for the first few days. Its composition is very similar to rabbit's milk, containing 74 percent water, 12.4 percent protein, 8.6 percent fat and virtually no carbohydrates.

Surrogate parents

Domesticated doves or pigeons can be used as surrogates. The softbill eggs should be synchronized to hatch at approximately the same time as those of the surrogate—to ensure that the chick receives the all important crop milk—although experiments have shown that milk will still be produced up to about 2 days before and/or after the surrogate expects the egg to hatch.

Hand rearing

Unfortunately, hand rearing pigeons and doves from day 1 is an uncertain process. The difficulty does not seem to be in providing the correct nutrition, but rather, in supplying the correct bacteria that will populate the gut and thus enable the bird to properly digest its food. It may be that the parents' saliva plays an important role, as I suspect it does in helping newly hatched insectivores to digest their food. But it is difficult to be certain, and this is clearly a subject in need of further research. Chicks that have been fed by their parents for the first seven days, however, are fairly easy to hand feed thereafter.

Hand rearing can be attempted as follows: for the first 30 percent of the fledging period, feed the chick with an artificial crop milk. This can be made by mixing together equal parts of an oral electrolyte (such as Pedialyte™) and premixed Isomil™ or SMA™. As the chick grows it will need a thicker diet. Puree some of the adult food and add it to the milk. Mix together, and if necessary dilute with water for a creamy paste.

Problems during Hand Feeding

Refusal to feed/defecate

The environmental temperature may be too low or the food may be too cold. A refusal to feed can also be caused by discomfort if the chick is unable to defecate, and it may need to be stimulated with something like a moistened cloth. Normally, feces should be produced fairly easily and without encouragement. But if problems occur, the fiber content of the diet may be too low. Add high fiber foods, such as pureed pumpkin, equal to about 10 percent of the whole volume.

Most softbills produce fecal sac droppings until approximately fledging time with soft adult droppings produced once the youngster has left the nest.

Aspiration

This is where solids or fluids are inhaled. It can occur if too much food has been delivered into the mouth or if the proper feeding response has not first been elicited. Equally, very small chicks are susceptible to aspiration after they have been fed: as the chick lays down, food can reflux back up the esophagus and into the mouth, from where it is aspirated.

If only a small amount of food has been aspirated, the bird may cough, sneeze, shake its head and gasp for air to clear the fluid from the trachea. If food has entered a lung or cannot be cleared from the trachea, the bird's breathing will become labored and a clicking or rasping sound may be heard. The bird can die immediately; or death may occur hours or days later from the effects of **aspiration pneumonia**. Your veterinarian can treat the pneumonia, but the outlook by this time is usually grave.

Sour crop

The crop should be empty, or very nearly so, at the beginning of every feed. It should be allowed to completely empty at least once every 24 hours. Feeding a bird while food remains in the crop may turn the residue bad. This is a common cause of death in hand-reared chicks and such accumulations must be quickly removed, otherwise slow gut transit time will result, leading to total gut stasis and death.

A length of soft rubber tubing can be used to syringe warm water into the crop. Gently massage the crop to break up any lumps of food, and use the syringe to remove the mixture; repeat the process until the fluid drawn from the crop is clear.

If the lumps of food are hard to remove, molasses mixed with equal parts of warm water may be fed to the chick; massaging the crop to assist the process, even quite hard residues can be dislodged and washed through the body with no ill-effects. Feed the molasses mixture for several feedings, or until the lumps of food have gone.

Once the crop is clear, 1 or 2 feedings of the normal volume should be attempted. Use a balanced electrolyte, such as Pedialyte™; or a "stage one" human baby food diet (fruit), mixed half and half with water. If the crop empties properly, feeding with the normal food can be resumed; but dilute the formula for the first few feeds until normal crop motility returns. If motility does not return, resume the crop-wash procedure.

Crop burn

If the food is too hot, the delicate tissue of the crop and esophagus can be burned. A scab may appear several days later on the skin covering the crop, and up to 4 days later leakage can be expected. Recovery may be assisted by a topical application of a vitamin E ointment, although mild burns should heal themselves.

In severe cases surgical repair may be necessary. If the affected area is fairly small, this is relatively easy in skilled hands. But a larger area of damaged tissue is harder to repair; and if the damage is considerable, insufficient tissue may remain to rebuild a viable esophagus. In such cases euthanasia must be considered.

Deformed beaks

Poor hand-feeding techniques are often blamed for such problems, even though very experienced hand feeders also produce affected birds. In some cases the damage can be caused by defects in the bird, the incubation or the parents' diet. If detected early enough, a deformed beak can be corrected simply by manipulating it into its proper position several times a day. The key is to do this when the beak is still very young and malleable.

References

Fox, Dr. N. *Understanding the Bird of Prey*. Hancock House Publishers, 1995.

Harvey, R. *Practical Incubation*. Second edition. Hancock House Publishers, 1993.

Kuehler, C. and Good, J. "Artificial incubation of bird eggs at the Zoological Society of San Diego." *International Zoo Yearbook*. 1990. 29: 118–136.

11

Ailments

An excellent diet, clean drinking water and a stress-free and sanitary environment will lead to a healthy collection. All things being equal softbills can be long-lived in captivity: more than 10 years for some hummingbirds, 20 years for certain thrushes and 50 years or more for the larger hornbills.

But sooner or later you will encounter a sick bird and its prompt diagnosis and treatment are often vital for a recovery. If the softbills are looked after by different people, simply noticing a sick bird can be a problem; but if they are cared for by the same person, even tiny changes in their behavior and appearance can be spotted. Any changes can be critical, since birds will do their best to mask signs of disease. In the wild, they may otherwise be more easily eaten or picked on by flock members in status checks.

Treatment

When a bird looks poorly it is often difficult to decide on the best course of action. For the very small and delicate softbills merely catching them to facilitate a veterinary examination can be extremely stressful. Generally if the subject looks only very slightly off-color, leaving it alone, adding a probiotic treatment to its food and offering an infrared lamp is usually all the medicine it needs—provided there are no external pressures such as violence or persecution from another. (See Ailments—probiotics.)

But if the condition persists for more than a day or so, or if there are any obvious symptoms, seek immediate veterinary advice. Possible warning signs are bloodstained or loose droppings, appetite loss, inactivity, sitting on or near the ground, half-open eyes, fluffed-up feathers, a marked deterioration of feather condition, paralysis or labored breathing—characterized by tail-bobbing.

A sick bird may be infectious and will need to be separated from the others and kept warm, preferably in an incubator, or a quarantine cage with heat, at a temperature of 86°F (30°C). Alternatively a thermostatically controlled hospital cage can be purchased or a simple homemade version, employing an infrared lamp, is often suitable. Or an infrared lamp can be fixed to the cage front, providing warmth but also allowing the bird to retreat if it gets too hot. A low perch should be provided and positioned so that the bird cannot defecate in its food or water; harmful bacteria or viruses may be present in the droppings and reingesting them will only hamper a treatment. In the warm hospital cage, food and water dishes dry out very quickly and should to be replaced frequently.

If a visit to the veterinarian's office is required, a small portable incubator, designed to plug into a car's cigarette lighter, is the ideal means of transport. Otherwise a cooler containing a hot-water bottle works equally well, with the bird's feet protected from scalding by a thick layer of towels. The veterinarian will examine the softbill and if necessary take various samples such as blood, droppings or swabs from the throat or cloaca. These will then be examined in the laboratory and a suitable treatment should recommend itself.

Hygiene

We all know that prevention is better than cure; but something about human nature allows us to neglect the fundamental principles of hygiene, until it is too late.

Yeast and bacteria are everywhere in the environment and it is practically impossible to remove them. A healthy bird can fight off many of the pathogenic organisms it encounters, but a bird that has been immune-compromised (by poor nutrition, stress, disease, molt, old age or growth) may become ill. And if levels of bacteria or yeast are high enough, even a fully fit and healthy bird can be overwhelmed. It is therefore important to minimize the effects of such organisms with good hygiene practices, the value of which should never be underestimated.

Bacteria

Normal flora: these are bacteria that live in and on animals and are not harmful; they can even block pathogens.

Opportunistic pathogens: bacteria out of balance or in the wrong place. Not normally a problem except in the immune-compromised.

Pathogens: disease-causing bacteria which invade and cause damage.

Sources of pathogenic bacteria and yeast

Food

Contamination can be caused by poor handling practices since there are bacteria, such as some strains of *E. coli*, that are harmless to us, but pathogenic for most softbills. Wash your hands thoroughly before preparing food.

Prepare moist foods fresh each day. Store dry foods in closed containers to protect them from vermin and help prevent oxidation. Keep a clean scoop in each container to fill food dishes; do not dip dishes into the main food source in case the dish is contaminated.

Position food and water dishes so that perching birds cannot defecate in them. Provide fresh food and water at least once a day. Clean and disinfect food dishes every day; keep in use two sets of dishes so that clean and dry ones are always available. Clean and disinfect water dishes every week; and scrub them with a brush each day to prevent the accumulation of a biofilm, a haven for potentially harmful bacteria.

Frozen food can be contaminated if allowed to thaw out over a prolonged period. Keep food refrigerated while thawing or use a microwave oven.

Water

Water pipes can harbor bacteria, especially PVC pipes, and it is a good idea to run the water for 2 minutes before use. Also, periodically clean or replace the screen in the water tap.

Environmental

Contamination of the environment is a prime cause of disease. Soiled perches, accumulations of dried feces, poor ventilation and rotting food all invite disease, and all are relatively easy to prevent. Cleaning agents such as bleach, Roccal™, the generic chlorhexidine products (like Nolvasan™), and the phenol disinfectants like Tektrol™ can all be used for disease prevention and control.

Disinfectants

Disinfectants become less effective when mixed with organic material, soaps and detergents; it is therefore important to thoroughly clean and rinse surfaces before disinfection. Most disinfectants take up to 15 minutes to work effectively; ideally surfaces should be sprayed with the disinfectant and left to soak before being rinsed.

Cleaning and disinfecting the aviary and bird room is essential following a disease outbreak. But it is best not to start cleaning until the birds have been treated for several days. By this time the organisms being shed into the environment will have been greatly reduced; and if the aviary is again cleaned and disinfected at the end of the treatment period, it should become totally free of the disease.

All disinfectants have their good and bad points and must be used knowledgeably in the avian environment.

Bleach: kills virtually all organisms except avian tuberculosis. It produces fumes that are quickly toxic to birds; and it is not effective in the presence of organic material such as feces or food remains.

Synthetic phenols: kill virtually all organisms and are quite effective in the presence of organic material. They remain effective (and toxic) for several days; birds should be kept away from recently cleaned surfaces.

Ammonias: kill most organisms except avian tuberculosis, *Candida* and aspergillosis; and they are not effective in the presence of organic material.

Droppings and Their Diagnostic Value

It is important that you become familiar with the normal appearance of your birds' droppings, since changes in them can provide an early warning of many problems. Even if the droppings appear normal, a fecal examination every 6 months by your veterinarian is recommended to help detect problems such as worms, coccidiosis and candidiasis.

Collect several fresh stools from the same cage or aviary and refrigerate them in an old 35-mm film canister. Date the canister and give it to your veterinarian as soon as possible. Do not freeze the sample and be sure to record the test results on the bird's record.

Birds urinate and defecate at the same time; waste from the urinary tract and gastrointestinal tract is deposited in the cloaca before being released from the body. The dropping is made up of 3 parts:

Feces: this is the unusable solid waste from food and is the central, major part of the dropping. Its color and consistency can be affected by diet, with pelletized foods often producing a more brownish appearance. Changes in color generally point to infection, or disease of the liver or pancreas. Very loose stools or diarrhea can be caused by spoiled food, a sudden change of diet, intestinal infection, parasites, stress, egg binding, organ disease, excessive antibiotic use, or the ingestion of poison or a foreign object.

Urine: most softbills produce a relatively large amount of urine because their diets are often high in fruits and vegetables. An increased urine output may occur with stress and a decreased output can indicate dehydration. Urine analysis is not commonly done for birds but is useful when urinary tract infections, kidney disease, diabetes and even heavy-metal poisoning are suspected.

Urates (Uric Acid): the urate portion of the dropping typically sits on or around the feces. It is powdery and normally white or white-beige in color; it is usually affected by liver disease.

Laboratory Analyses

Under the microscope a stool sample can be examined for the presence of internal parasites such as worms and protozoa. Potentially pathogenic bacteria, yeast and fungi may be detected in a culture. And an acid fast test can be done to identify acid fast bacteria such as *Mycobacterium avium*, the main cause of avian tuberculosis.

Botulism

Any decaying protein is a potential source of *Clostridium botulinum*. It can grow in any anaerobic environment such as soil or intestine, but most frequently it is found in rotten meat. For the aviculturist, maggots fed infected meat are the main source of the bacteria; it is therefore essential that maggots are thoroughly cleaned before use. (See Diets—maggots.) The toxin produced by this bacteria affects the nervous system—the bird's legs extend backwards, parallel with the tail, and its body is paralyzed, unable to move except to flop along on its belly.

Botulism can affect all of your birds and once they start to show any symptoms, successful treatment is unlikely. Losses can be high and the best course of action is to treat those that have not yet developed any symptoms with a solution of Epsom salts (hydrated magnesium sulphate). Given orally this will hopefully purge the body of the clostridial bacteria and protect it from absorbing a fatal dose of the toxin. Mix water and Epsom salts in a 50:50 ration; using a tube, fill the crop twice daily for 5 days. Even with this treatment recovery is uncertain, and because of the associated risks, I normally avoid maggots all together.

A vaccine developed for mink (Botumink) has been used at the Denver Zoo in Colorado, apparently very successfully and with no side effects. To date, over 1,000 doses have been administered to birds. The vaccine can be obtained from United Vaccines Inc., P.O. Box 44220, Madison, WI, 53744. (*The Quill*, 1996.)

Aspergillosis

This is a fungal disease predominantly of the lower respiratory tract and in most cases is caused by *Aspergillus fumigatus*. Throughout their environment, birds are continually exposed to the *Aspergillus* spores, and it is only under certain conditions that the fungal agents become pathogenic. Death is normally the result and although the fungus can be rapidly fatal, its development is usually slow and insidious.

The growth of mold in the bird's environment should be avoided in an effort to keep the number of airborne spores to a minimum. Poor ventilation coupled with dampness, old food, accumulations of droppings or decaying vegetation will all encourage the growth of *Aspergillus* and other fungi; and if the softbills are already weakened by disease, stress or malnutrition they will surely succumb.

Frequently aspergillosis is not apparent until well established. It takes over the air passages, mainly the lungs and air sacs, and affected birds often appear short of breath after moderate exertion. They will likely exhibit open-mouthed and noisy breathing, and may experience a change in voice as the syrinx (the avian equivalent of the larynx) becomes affected. Typically such birds look rather dejected and are much less active than usual, especially toward the end of their illness.

Unfortunately, an accurate diagnosis tends to come from an autopsy, although it is possible to identify aspergillosis by using exploratory surgery. If the disease is confirmed, all other birds in the building should be monitored carefully for any of the telltale symptoms, especially labored, open-mouthed breathing. If the birds look normal but you suspect aspergillosis, make them fly the full length of their aviary and watch their breathing once they have landed. The accommodation should be thoroughly cleaned in an attempt to eradicate the fungal spores: Nolvasan™, bleach and phenols are all effective. To help prevent future outbreaks, cleaning practices and the ventilation system should also be examined.

Aspergillosis can be cured with drugs such as Flucytosine and especially Itraconazole. X-rays can be used to monitor the disease; and if treated early enough, the outlook can be surprisingly good. However, reinfection may occur fairly easily if the bird is subjected to any of the causative factors mentioned above.

Candidiasis (*Candida albicans*)

This is another type of fungus (a yeast), affecting mostly the upper digestive tract and the mouth. In the early stages, there are no symptoms whatsoever, although the fungus may be detected during a fecal examination. *Candida* live normally in a healthy bird, but can become pathogenic if the gut flora is upset. Malnutrition, vitamin A deficiency or prolonged antibiotic treatment can create gaps in the body's defenses and may result in overgrowth. Indeed, giving a precautionary treatment of Nystatin following prolonged antibiotic therapy is highly beneficial.

Opening the mouth of an infected bird will normally reveal the whitish, cottage cheeselike masses of fungus. In advanced cases candidiasis can prevent the bird from eating, and force-feeding may be necessary. The softbill may even breathe with its mouth partly open and tongue protruding; this will put at risk others in the vicinity and the infected bird should be removed to separate accommodation. To help confine the outbreak further, all of the food and water dishes should be thoroughly cleaned and disinfected since it is through them that a *Candida* infection is often spread.

The disease can be treated with an antibiotic prescribed by your veterinarian. Most *Candida* are susceptible to Nystatin which is frequently used to treat upper-gastrointestinal candidiasis. There are few side effects and Nystatin is not absorbed from the gastrointestinal tract following oral administration. Treat orally for 5 days (once daily 1 ml Nystatin/400 g of bird). In severe cases where the mouth is full of the fungus, paint the Nystatin directly onto the affected areas with an artist's brush.

Nectivores that are being hand reared can be susceptible to yeast infections, and Nystatin may be added to their formula on a prophylactic basis—consult your veterinarian. Vitamin A supplementation may also be helpful.

Salmonella

In a well-kept aviary this disease is uncommon, although since it can be introduced by rats and mice all softbills are vulnerable. It is insidious and difficult, if not impossible, to eliminate; *Salmonella* likes moist environments and fecal contamination. Newly imported birds are most often infected and in their weakened state succumb rapidly.

Affected birds look depressed, fluffed-up, listless and tend to produce diarrhea. Laboratory work will be required to establish the existence of *Salmonella*, its type and recommended antibiotic treatment. Meanwhile the subject will be dehydrating, and the loss of fluids must be replaced until medication begins to take effect. In a small bird, dehydration is normally rapid and death occurs before the laboratory tests can be completed.

However, the most modern electrolytic supplements may help sustain a sick bird until the medication starts to work. As well as electrolytes, these products include long-chain glucose polymers (to supply energy) and nutrients such as proteins and vitamins. Poly-Aid is perhaps one of the most advanced supplements of this kind; and although it is not available in the United States, information can be obtained from Vetafarm Europe Ltd, 5 Cossack Square, Nailsworth, Glos, Gl6 0DB, U.K.

On occasions where *Salmonella* can be predicted—such as when receiving a shipment of birds from the wild—a precautionary antibiotic treatment may prevent large losses, especially in smaller birds that cannot wait for laboratory tests to be done. Administering a broad-spectrum antibiotic (such as Terramycin or Aureomycin) or a probiotic from the first day of quarantine can prove very advantageous. Consult your veterinarian. (See Probiotics and below.)

Antibiotics as a Prophylactic

It is extremely important to realize that using any antibiotic as a prophylactic is not ideal, and must be done rarely and with the consent of your veterinarian. Indiscriminate or prolonged use can result in overgrowth of nonsusceptible bacteria; and bacteria can become resistant, making future treatment much more difficult.

However, softbills imported from the wild can be infected with *Salmonella* and other diseases; and a broad-spectrum antibiotic can prevent large losses, especially in small or delicate species. I have found such medications to be worthwhile for many shipments of sunbird-sized birds when used from day 1 of the quarantine. Consult your veterinarian.

Escherichia coli

This is another type of bacteria which is normally treatable. On occasion, however, it can lead to enteritis (inflammation of the intestine) which can be fatal. While *E. coli* exists in the digestive system of mammals, including people, some varieties (but not all) can be dangerous to birds and can be transmitted by dirty hands.

Hygiene is therefore important in the food preparation area and especially when hand feeding chicks.

Most birds have predominantly gram-positive gut flora, while mammals and reptiles have gram-negative flora, like *E. coli*. However, there is always some *E. coli* in any bird and it can even be normal flora in ground feeders. Therefore, certain birds such as ducks, ratites and chickens have mainly gram-negative bacteria.

Birds infected with *E. coli* often retain a fairly normal appetite but are unable to perch. Expect to see fluffed up feathers and loose droppings, with pasted urates and feces on the vent; greenish diarrhea may indicate enteritis. New arrivals are particularly at risk since they may have experienced a diet change and be suffering from a digestive disturbance. And anything that upsets the normal gut flora—including excessive or indiscriminate antibiotic use—may invite problems.

Following laboratory tests, a suitable antibiotic will be prescribed by your veterinarian. Treatment is usually successful leading to a complete recovery.

Coccidiosis

This is a protozoan disease—caused by single-cell organisms—and severely infected birds lose their appetite, look miserable, become emaciated and produce green diarrhea. Usually though, mildly infected birds show no symptoms and microscopic analysis of their droppings is needed to confirm the diagnosis. Indeed without such an examination many cases of coccidiosis would go undetected.

In themselves, mild infections are more of a nuisance than a threat to life. But the very young, old, sick or stressed are at risk to severe complications, and it is important to treat affected birds.

Treatment can be with a sulfonamide (such as sulfadimidine or sulfaquinoxaline) or amprolium prescribed by your veterinarian. Amprolium (trade name Corid) is a common coccidiostat: 4.8 ml/3.77 liters of water, offered as the sole source of drinking water for five days (3.77 liters = 1 U.S. gallon or 0.83 Imperial gallon). Treatment should be repeated 14 days after the end of the first treatment. And then once the second treatment is complete, 2 fecal examinations (14 days apart) will be needed to confirm a cure.

Pseudotuberculosis (Yersiniosis)

This can be an extremely potent disease spread by mice and rats. The softbill will look under-the-weather for a day or so before death. Equally, sufferers can die after several days of weight loss and gradual deterioration.

The disease can be verified by an autopsy with damage to the liver similar to that of tuberculosis. Antibiotics may help affected birds, although a return to full health is very rare since the rapid course of the disease makes early detection unlikely.

Worms

The eggs of these parasites can be detected during a fecal examination, provided the worms are laying eggs at the time. The effects of worms are increasingly debilitating and it is a good idea to treat the entire collection on a prophylactic basis every 6 months.

Treatment is easy, using one of the proprietary wormers based on the drugs albendazole, mebendazole, thiabendazole or fenbendazole. Panacur is the trade name of a commonly available wormer based on fenbendazole and can be obtained from a veterinarian.

One treatment alone can be useless: it is very important to repeat the treatment 14 days after the first one is complete, to help prevent reinfection. In addition, the aviary should be thoroughly cleaned and disinfected, and the substrate disinfected or replaced. This should clear away the parasites' eggs or host animals.

Constantly using the same wormer can lead to resistant worms. It is therefore important to change the wormer every year, rotating between products that use different drugs.

Caution: albendazole may be toxic to some species. Veterinarians at the San Diego Zoo and San Diego Wild Animal Park found that albendazole may be toxic to keas, *Nestor notabilis*; southern speckled pigeons, *Columba guinea phaenota*; and pink-spotted fruit doves, *Ptilinopus perlatus*. (Ilse H. Stalis, DVM et al. 1995.)

Tapeworms (cestodes) cause obstruction and compete with the body for nutrients in the gut. An infected bird passes the worm eggs in its droppings which in turn are eaten by an insect. When that insect is then eaten by another bird the tapeworm can grow to maturity and repeat the cycle. Insectivorous birds are naturally most at risk although at some time in their lives the vast majority of softbills eat insects, and so all should be protected.

Roundworms (nematodes): many species drain blood or impair gut function. Worm eggs are mostly passed directly from bird to bird in the droppings, and are swallowed as birds feed on the ground or on soiled food. Some roundworms have a larval stage that crawls onto vegetation to infect the next host.

Capillaria (nematodes): also known as gapeworm, these tiny, threadlike parasites infect the lungs and trachea, causing respiratory problems, and an increased risk of secondary infection. Affected birds may cough and shake their heads in an effort to remove the parasite.

Mites and Lice

Feather mites and feather lice can cause irritation, scaling and feather plucking leading to damaged or patchy plumage. Most mites and lice are external parasites and can be easily treated using a proprietary remedy. Powders containing pyrethrin, rotinone or malathion are effective, and treatment should be repeated after about 2 weeks.

Apply liberally, particularly around the vent, neck and under the wings. Take care to shield the bird's head, since inhalation of the powder can cause respiratory damage. Pyrethrins are the safest.

Ivermectin is also very good for the treatment of external parasites, although there is no specific product license for avian use, since it was developed for large animals. It must therefore be used completely at your own risk; but having said that, it is in fact very safe and effective. Ivermectin comes in different forms which must all be diluted for use on birds.

The British veterinarian Alan Jones, MRCVS, uses the 1 percent cattle injection, diluted 1 in 9 to give a 0.1 percent preparation. Sterile water can be used to make a suspension for immediate use, otherwise the diluent must be propylene glycol. The medication is then applied to the bird's skin to treat external parasites; and because it is absorbed into the bloodstream, internal parasites (such as intestinal worms) can also be treated in this way. Equally, oral administration or injection can be used: 0.2 ml diluted Ivermectin/ 1 kg of bodyweight. (1996 *Bird Keeper.*)

Red mites are more troublesome than other ectoparasites since they are able to live away from the body, secreted in the aviary's crevices and in nest boxes. They come out at night and live by sucking blood from the bird, causing anemia and death in severe cases.

As well as treating the softbill, its aviary will have to be thoroughly cleaned and disinfected along with all of the fixtures and fittings. It is not sufficient to simply leave the aviary empty for a period, since this particular parasite can live without food for several months.

Care should be taken if wild birds' nests are used to help stimulate captive breeding. They are sometimes infested with red mites, and must be disinfected and thoroughly dried before use.

Air-sac mites are internal parasites which live in the bird's respiratory system. Affected birds often wheeze and may show signs of respiratory distress after gentle exercise. Treatment is usually with an injectable drug such as Ivermectin. And repeat doses are needed as recent research has shown that single doses do not eliminate the parasites.

Bumblefoot

Although more often associated with waterfowl and birds of prey, softbills are also vulnerable to bumblefoot, particularly terrestrial species. The condition is caused by an infection, mainly from an injury or abrasion on the foot. It is commonly the result of floor coverings or perches that are too hard for the species concerned; or perches of a uniform diameter, like doweling, can cause a similar injury. A soft, clean, variable surface such as peat moss, grass or fresh perches will help prevent bumblefoot.

Pittas, wagtails, chats, robins and wading birds should all be monitored for any foot problems. Persistently holding one foot up, apparently in some discomfort, is usually the first sign of an infection. And if an examination reveals swelling on the undersurface of the foot, veterinary advice should be sought immediately.

Abscesses may need to be lanced and your veterinarian may use an antibiotic locally and internally. In advanced cases, bumblefoot can be exceedingly difficult to eradicate and surgery is likely. Curing the condition often depends on very early detection, and good observation is vital.

On occasions when veterinary help has not been available, I have treated minor abrasions by cleaning them with hydrogen peroxide and applying an antibiotic ointment, such as Mycitracin™ or Neosporin™. This seems to be a good first aid measure, although veterinary advice should always be sought as soon as possible.

Gangrene

This is the death of tissue caused by an absence of the blood supply. It can be the result of frostbite, severe fractures, dietary deficiencies or dried food that has been allowed to encase a toe. But the most common causes of gangrene are tightly fitting leg bands and fibers (such as nesting material) tangled around the leg or foot.

Good observation should detect the problem as affected birds continuously favor one foot over the other. Recovery is usually complete, provided the constriction is soon removed. If this is not done, the foot or toe will come off.

Frostbite is also a fairly common cause of this type of injury, and a frost-free shelter is essential. Perch heaters in the flight will offer a measure of protection, although on their own they are no substitute for a proper house. (See Housing—perch heaters.)

Iron-Storage Disease

As part of evolution, animals adapt to environmental conditions and local foods. Where foods are low in iron, for example, species tend to develop particularly efficient mechanisms for iron absorption and utilization. Certain species are therefore vulnerable to excessive amounts of iron in their diet.

This disease was first discovered in the hill mynah (*Gracula religiosa*) and birds of paradise. Studies showed that birds of paradise can absorb up to 90 percent of all the iron in their diet. Barbets, quetzals, touracos, tanagers and toucans are also susceptible to iron-storage disease and probably benefit from low-iron diets. But in the case of toucans, they should only be given low-iron pellets that do not contain propylene glycol, since this can be fatal for all toucans, especially the large black species (Jennings 1996).

Low levels of iron are considered to be less than 100 ppm (parts per million) with less than 70 ppm being ideal. Excessive amounts are stored in body tissues—especially the liver which is damaged in the process—eventually leading to hemosiderosis and perhaps hemochromatosis.

One of the first signs of iron-storage poisoning is a reduced ability to fly. This is caused by a swollen abdomen which is often distended with fluid called ascites. Labored breathing and muscle wasting may also be seen.

Even if the bird shows none of these symptoms, the liver damage caused by iron-storage poisoning can affect breeding. Proteins essential for egg development are no longer produced and breeding does not occur.

There is not a specific treatment; but you should put the birds on a low-iron diet and avoid large amounts of dried fruits which can contribute to the disease. Removing blood may be helpful, but normally the bird will deteriorate over several months and die.

Rickets

This is a disease characterized by soft or defective bones. It is caused by a lack of calcium or vitamin D_3, and particularly affects the fast-growing skeleton of a chick. Although serious when established, rickets is easily prevented by sprinkling a multivitamin and mineral supplement on the rearing food.

The body can also obtain vitamin D_3 by natural synthesis, if it is given access to direct sunlight or full-spectrum Vitalites™ positioned within a foot or 2 of the bird—no matter how much calcium is supplemented, it will not be absorbed and used by the body unless there is sufficient D_3. The calcium:phosphorus ratio is also important and must be in balance at about 2:1.

Supplementation is especially important for insectivores: such chicks have to live purely on insects for the first several weeks of their lives, until they are old enough to feed themselves and eat the nutritionally superior adult diet. Omnivores, on the other hand, may have to live on live food for only a week or so, receiving the more balanced adult food soon after.

In practice therefore, insectivores tend to be more susceptible to rickets, although it is prudent to feed a multivitamin and mineral supplement to all chicks.

Night Frights

After nightfall, vermin or thunder and lightning can terrify even the most steady and established birds. And in blind panic they can collide with the wire mesh or the numerous other obstacles. The provision of a night light, to simulate moonlight, will considerably reduce such accidents which can be fatal. The birds can also feed after dark, allowing them to maintain vital body reserves in low temperatures. (See night lights on page 25.)

Victims of night frights frequently suffer head injuries although little is usually seen from a casual examination. Feathers may be slightly ruffled but blood is normally absent from the scalp and damage to the skull is only obvious from within. Blood may be present, however, if death is caused by striking a sharp object or an attack from another.

As with all fatalities, an autopsy by your veterinarian is recommended for a fuller explanation of the cause of death. During the examination, the skin of the scalp may be peeled back to reveal the semi-transparent skull, through which is often seen a patch of blue-red hemorrhage. If the skull is opened, blood may be seen to have penetrated the bone of the skull itself. This cannot happen with bleeding produced by a burst blood vessel in the brain or disease of the arteries: the membranes that cover the brain are quite strong and capable of confining cerebral bleeding to the brain surface. The presence of blood in the cranial bones is therefore proof that the hemorrhage was caused by a blow to the head.

Probiotics—A Prophylactic

Probiotics are a mixture of essential amino acids, vitamins and the beneficial microorganisms found in a bird's gut. These supplements are familiar ingredients in the hand-rearing regimes of psittacines, and others, being used to create the gut flora necessary for a chick's normal digestion; they are also useful for re-establishing the gut flora in an adult bird following prolonged antibiotic therapy. But less well known are the important roles probiotics can play in helping birds that may be sick or vulnerable to infection.

Within a healthy gut is found both beneficial and potentially harmful bacteria. The beneficial bacteria compete for binding sites on the gut wall and produce inhibiting substances to limit the influence of pathogens, such as *Salmonella* and *Escherichia coli*. If, however, a bird is put under stress the conditions in its gut may change.

Shipping a bird induces considerable stress, especially when it has been caught from the wild and sent many thousands of miles. It will invariably arrive exhausted and vulnerable to any pathogens it may encounter. Added to which, when unpacked into its new environment, the bird may meet unfamiliar microorganisms and will almost certainly experience a diet change. Such stresses will favor the harmful bacteria of the gut which can multiply and have a debilitating effect, dampening the bird's morale and keenness to feed. Even if none of the vital organs is affected, the softbill can very quickly go downhill, so an attempt to eradicate the invading bacteria is normally made.

Samples are taken, cultured and tested with various antibiotics. These sensitivity tests identify the most effective drug which is then administered. The problem is that by the time the laboratory tests have been completed, the bird may have died or passed the point of no return. Equally, an entire shipment of softbills may have to get progressively sicker as they wait a few vital days for the laboratory analysis of an autopsy.

A bird whose illness is difficult to quickly diagnose may be fed a probiotic treatment, which at the very least will act as a stop-gap until a perhaps more potent (antibiotic) drug can be identified. If any parts of the gut are disturbed, a probiotic can affect them ahead of an invading pathogen. The spread of the bacteria would then be slowed, giving the body time to stabilize itself and muster its own defenses.

If a bird appears healthy but is considered at risk from disease or the potentially damaging effects of stress, it should be fed a probiotic as a precautionary measure. In this way a pathogen can be treated before it gets a chance to inflict any real harm.

Common Ailments

The following table summarizes only the ailments mentioned in this chapter, and therefore represents just a few of the possible health care questions you may have about your birds. It is merely a quick reference guide to some of the more common ailments and cannot replace the expertise of your avian veterinarian. A trained diagnosis is essential before the proper treatment can be administered; and a consultation with your veterinarian is vital if a bird is sick.

Acknowledgments

I would like to thank Dr. Matt Dahlquist, DVM for correcting the text of this chapter, for offering many valuable suggestions and for his considerable help in its preparation.

References

Bird Keeper, January 1996 issue. IPC Magazines Ltd, London, England.
Jennings, J. 1996. Personal communication.
The Quill, Spring 1996. The Newsletter of the American Zoo and Aquarium Association's Avian Interest Group.
Stalis, Ilse H. DVM, Bruce A. Rideout, DVM, PhD, Jack L. Allen, DVM, Meg Sutherland-Smith, DVM. 1995. "Possible Albendazole Toxicity in Birds." 1995 Proceedings Joint Conference AAZV/WDA/AAWV.

Further Reading

Ritchie, B., Harrison, G. and Harrison, L. *Avian Medicine: Principles and Applications*. Florida. Wingers Publishing, Inc., 1994.

Common Ailments

Paralyzed body: legs extend backward. → **Botulism** → Treat survivors orally with Epsom salts to purge body of toxins.

Open-mouthed breathing. →

- **High environmental temperature** → Environmental temperature exceeds about 90°F (32.2°C). Improve ventiation/air-conditioning. Keep temperature below 85°F (29.5°C) for susceptible (higher altitude) species.
- **Aspergillosis (dejected appearance)** → Very early detection vital. Treatment with drugs such as Flucytosine and Itraconazole. Examine environmental hygiene and ventilation quality.
- **Candidiasis (low appetite)** → Vitamin A supplementation may be helpful. Treat orally with Nystatin for 5 days. Once daily, 1ml/400g of bird.

Depressed, fluffed-up, green diarrhea. → *Salmonella* → Require sensitivity tests to determine correct antibiotic treatment—veterinarian may permit use of broad-spectrum antibiotic.

Unable to perch. Loose droppings/greenish diarrhea. Often normal appetite. → *E. coli*

No symptoms in early stages; infection discovered by fecal exam. Severe infection: no appetite, miserable, emaciated, green diarrhea. → **Coccidiosis** → Sulfonamides or amprolium. Repeat treatment 14 days after the first one. Disinfect substrate and confirm cure with 2 fecal exams 14 days apart.

Death after 24 hours of looking poorly, or gradual weight loss and deterioration over several days before death. → **Pseudotuberculosis (Yersiniosis)** → Autopsy shows tuberculosis-like liver damage. Antibiotics may help affected birds, but unlikely. Eradicate mice and rats which are the principle carriers of the organism.

Symptoms	Condition	Treatment
Thin-bodied with good appetite. Gapeworm: coughing and shaking head trying to dislodge parasite.	Worms	Proprietary wormer based on albendazole, mebendazole, fenbendazole or thiabendazole. Repeat treatment 14 days after the first one. Disinfect substrate and confirm cure with 2 fecal exams 14 days apart.
Skin irritation, scaling and plucking.	Feather mites	Proprietary sprays or powders. Pyrethin powder is effective and particularly safe for the bird.
Respiratory distress and wheezing.	Air-sac mites	Injectable drug such as Ivermectin.
Holding the same foot up, apparently in discomfort.	Bumblefoot (swelling on undersurface of foot)	Your veterinarian may lance the abscess and treat with antibiotics internally and locally. Surgery is likely in severe cases and a cure often depends on very early detection.
	Gangrene (often foot or toes are constricted)	Remove the constriction (rings or entangled nesting fibers). Early detection should save the affected toe or foot. Otherwise foot or digit may be lost; also caused by severe fracture, dietary deficiency or frost bite.
Reduced ability to fly due to swollen abdomen; possible labored breathing and muscle wasting.	Iron-storage disease	Change to low-iron diet of less than 100 ppm, and preferably less than 70 ppm. Avoid large amounts of dried fruits which can contribute to the disease. Taking blood can help but death usually occurs after several months.
Frequent bone damage, even audible creaking of bones during movement.	Rickets	Neonates vulnerable, especially insectivores. Add vitamin and mineral supplement to rearing food until weaned.

12

Species Accounts

Order	Family

PASSERIFORMES
Corvidae — Crows, jays and magpies
Emberizidae — Tanagers
Emberizidae — Euphonias and chlorophonias
Emberizidae — Honeycreepers
Eurylaimidae — Broadbills
Icteridae — Oropendolas
Irenidae — Chloropsis
Irenidae — Fairy bluebirds
Muscicapidae — Old World flycatchers
Nectariniidae — Sunbirds and spiderhunters
Pittidae — Pittas
Pycnonotidae — Bulbuls
Sturnidae — Starlings and mynahs
Timaliidae — Pekin robin and silver-eared mesia
Timaliidae — Laughing thrushes
Turdidae — Shama and dhyal thrush
Zosteropidae — White eyes

CORACIIFORMES
Alcedinidae — Kingfishers and kookaburras
Bucerotidae — Hornbills
Coraciidae — Rollers
Meropidae — Bee eaters

PICIFORMES
Capitonidae — Barbets
Ramphastidae — Toucans, toucanets and aracaris

APODIFORMES
Trochilidae — Hummingbirds

CHARADRIIFORMES
Burhinidae — Thick-knees
Charadriidae — Lapwings and plovers
Jacanidae — Jacanas
Recurvirostridae — Avocets and stilts

COLUMBIFORMES
Columbidae — Fruit doves and fruit pigeons

CUCULIFORMES
Musophagidae — Touracos

GRUIFORMES
Rallidae — Rails, crakes, coots and gallinules

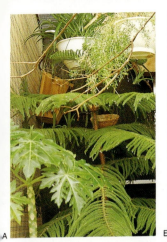
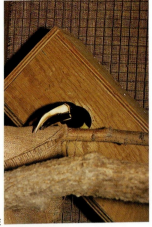
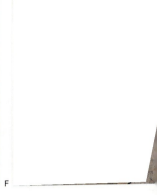
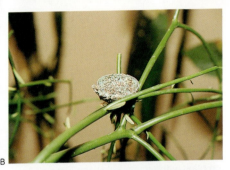
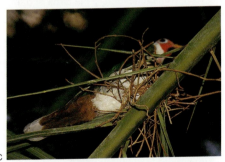
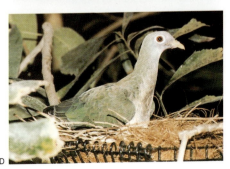

Breeding

A: A well-planted aviary helps provide seclusion for the breeding pair; and different types of nesting receptacles positioned in various locations will give the birds an important choice of nest sites. This aviary houses a pair of blue and yellow tanagers, *Thraupis bonariensis*. Nest sites include a cup-shaped wicker basket and two half open-fronted boxes, positioned at different heights.

B: Hummingbird nest platform made from half of a table tennis ball.

C: The egg being incubated by this male jambu fruit dove, *Ptilinopus jambu,* fell from the nest and smashed. A few months later the same pair was more successful when they accepted a wire mesh basket. Pictured in (D) is the female jambu fruit dove.

E: Black-necked aracaris, *Pteroglossus aracari*, nesting in a 5-foot (1.5m) tall box with a round entrance hole.

F: Parakeet-type box typically used by starlings and mynahs, seen here with grosbeak starlings, *Scissirostrum dubium*.

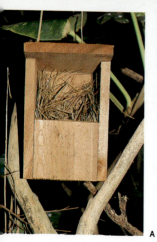
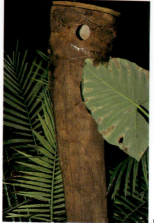
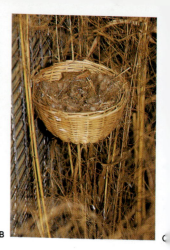
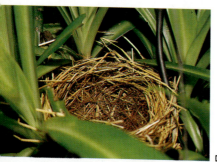
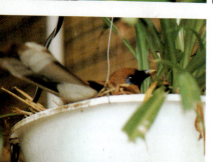

A. Half-open-fronted nest box, ideal for many small insectivores and builders of cup-shaped nests.
B: Palm log that has been excavated and nested in by a pair of black-headed woodpeckers, *Picus erythropygius*.
C: Wicker finch basket, nested in by a pair of bearded reedlings, *Panurus biarmicus*.
D: Spider plant in a hanging basket. Many softbills build their nests in planted hanging baskets. Irrigation tubes can be used to water the plant without disturbing the birds or damaging the nest. Note irrigation tube passing behind a liocichla nest.
E: Rufous laughing thrush, *Garrulax poecilorhynchus*, incubating in a planted hanging basket.
F: Nine-day-old black-naped fruit dove, *Ptilinopus melanospila*, on the edge of its nest basket a coconut fiber plant-pot liner.
G: An artificial rain system may help to define seasonal changes in the weather and promote breeding. It can also bring temporary relief to hot environments and is excellent for birds that are reluctant to bathe.

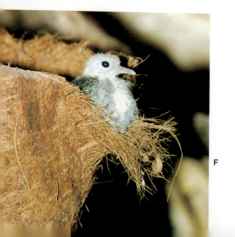
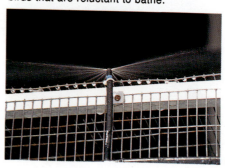

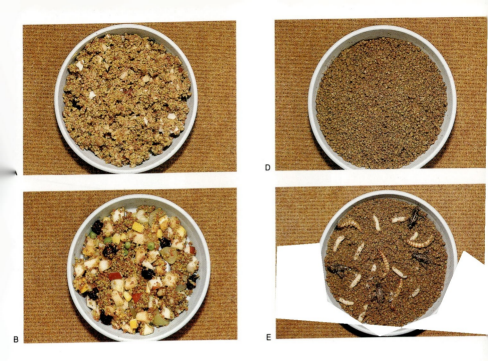

Diets

A: Basic appearance of Diets A, B and C for established birds, when using a small proprietary pellet such as Tropical Bits™.

B: Appearance of Diets A, B and C for newly purchased or imported birds that may not be feeding properly due to stress. The ingredients are exactly the same as in photo A, and in the same proportions; but to try to stimulate feeding, they are not mixed as thoroughly. Once the bird has started feeding normally, encourage it to eat the pellets (and therefore a more balanced diet) by mixing the ingredients together. In this way the diet for established birds (photo A) can be arrived at within about 2 weeks.

C: Diet G for standard insectivores.

D: Diet H for difficult insectivores. Stage 1: powdered proprietary softbill pellets.

E: Diet H, stage 2: livefood such as waxworms, giant mealworms and large crickets are soaked in nectar and placed on top of the powdered softbill pellets.

F: Diet H, stage 3: sprinkle with very finely chopped hard-boiled egg and thinly sliced pinkie mice (1mm thick).

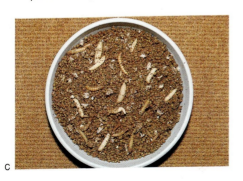
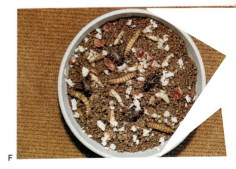

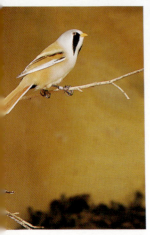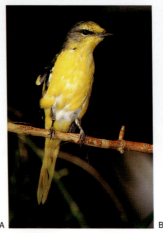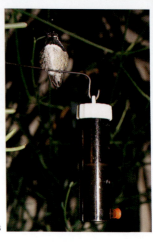

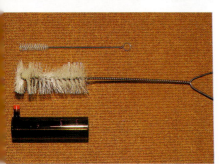

A: Diet G must be as fine and powdery as possible for small insectivores such as the Bearded reedling (male), *Panurus biarmicus*, and (B): Scarlet minivet (female), *Pericrocotus flammeus*.
C: Typical hummingbird feeder with a male Costa's hummingbird.
D: It is vital that nectar tubes are thoroughly cleaned every day. Use the correct brushes for both the tube and its spout.
E: Waxworms, mealworms and crickets come in various sizes, and it is important to select the one most suitable for your softbill.

Color Foods

Color foods are essential in the diets of the following softbills to maintain the vibrancy of their red, orange and yellow plumage.
F: Red-faced liocichla, *Liocichla phoenicea*.
G: Golden bush robin, *Tarsiger chrysaeus*.
H: Black-headed gonolek, *Laniarius erythrogaster*.
I: Andean cock-of-the-rock (male), *Rupicola peruviana*.

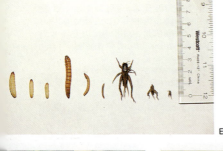

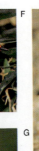
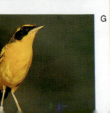
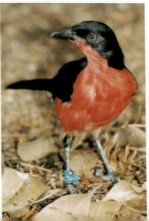
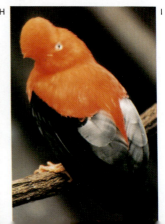

Ailments

A: A very sick looking male scarlet minivet, *Pericrocotus flammeus*: fluffed-up, eyes closed and drooping wings.

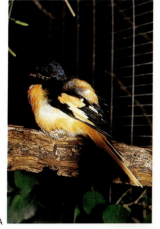

Nutrition

B: Newly imported female scarlet minivet. She had probably not had a bath for weeks and became saturated after over-bathing. This is particularly common for newly imported birds and especially dangerous for specimens released into enclosures with deep or running water. Such birds are easily swept away, and should first be allowed to bathe in shallow water to help revive their waterproofing. But even with established birds, bathing accidents can still occur; and in enclosures with dangerous watercourses, offering a dish of water beside the food is recommended, as has been done in (C) for a speckled mousebird, *Colius striatus*.

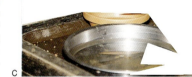

Housing

D: Breeding aviaries framed with 1 in. x 1 in. aluminum tubing. (Off-exhibit facility at Sedgwick County Zoo, Kansas.)
E: A feeding hatch allows dishes to be replaced quickly and keeps escapes to a minimum.
F: Some of the author's softbill aviaries in England.

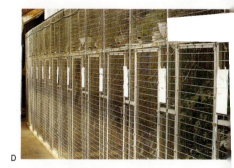

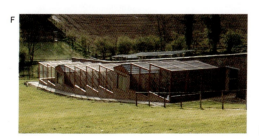

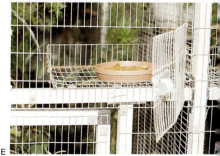

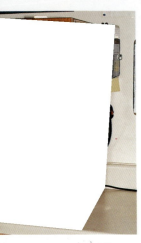 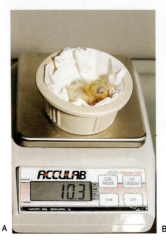 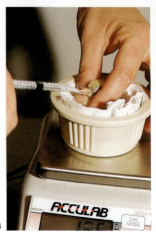

Incubation and Hand Rearing

A: A small Humidaire™ incubator
B: One-day-old pigeon. Monitoring a chick's weight throughout the hand-rearing process can provide the earliest warning of problems. Also, weighing the chick both before and after feedings, can help measure the consumption of minute amounts of food.

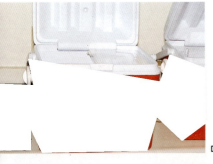

C: 1cc syringe used to feed a 2-day-old pigeon.
D: A portable incubator that can use mains power or be plugged into the cigarette lighter of a car.
E: White-tailed jays, *Cyanocorax mystacalis*. For the first few days, keeping chicks separated can help you monitor their progress and control disease.
F: Sulawesi king starlings, *Basilornis celebensis*—12 days old. As chicks grow older and stronger, keeping them together in a "creche" environment can help imprint them on each other rather than on you. (Continued next page.)

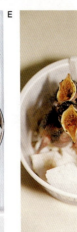 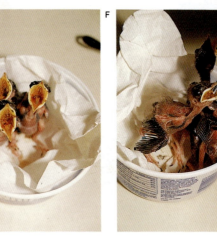

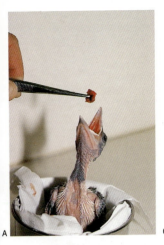
A

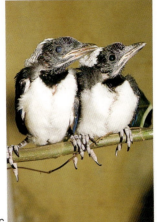
C

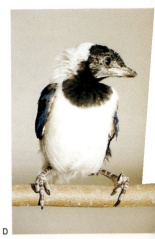
D

Opposite page:
G: Sulawesi king starlings—12 days old—being fed with tweezers.

A: White-tailed jay being fed with tweezers.
B: White-tailed jay being syringe fed.
C: Young white-tailed jays.
D: Young white-tailed jay with a foot defect. Such injuries may be caused during the hand-rearing process by incorrect or no substrate: help prevent leg and foot damage by using surfaces that the feet can grip onto from day 1.
E: African black crakes, *Porzana flavirostra*—4 days old—pictured feeding on finely chopped, hard-boiled egg, chopped waxworms and Tropical Bits™ (a tiny proprietary pellet). Members of the rail family are sub-precocial and should be offered food for the first several days.
F: Recently hatched pigeon feeding from inverted baby bottle nipple.
G: Five photo series, parent reared white-collared kingfisher, *Halcyon chloris*. First photo: 2 days old, continued next page.

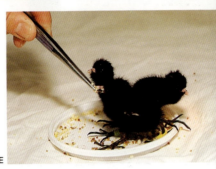
E

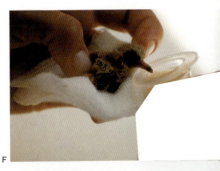
F

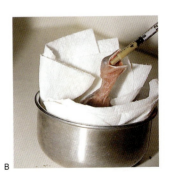
B

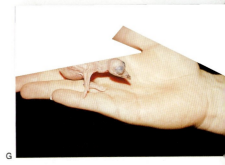
G

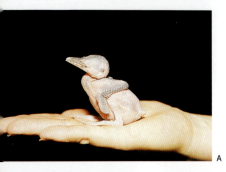

Five photo series, parent reared white-collared kingfisher, *Halcyon chloris*. (s/s female)

A: Second photo: 8 days old.
B: Third photo: 15 days old.
C: Fourth photo: (Front view) 4 months old.
D: Fifth photo: (Back view) 4 months old.

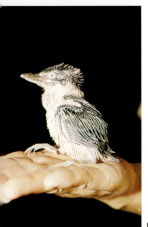
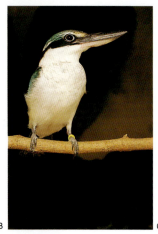
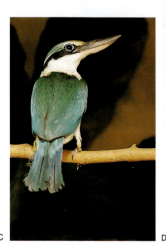

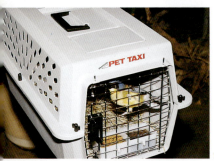

Catching and Handling

E: Small mammal carrying boxes are suitable for softbills and are accepted by airlines for domestic flights. It is advisable to provide food and water for all journeys; and to prevent the water from spilling out, sponge can be inserted in the dish.
F: The author uses both hands to restrain the body and the feet of a female Montezuma oropendola, *Psarocolius montezuma*.
G: The author demonstrates how to safely handle a small bird with one hand.

Photos: Renata Tramontana-Vince

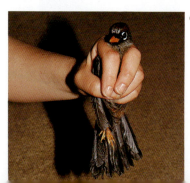

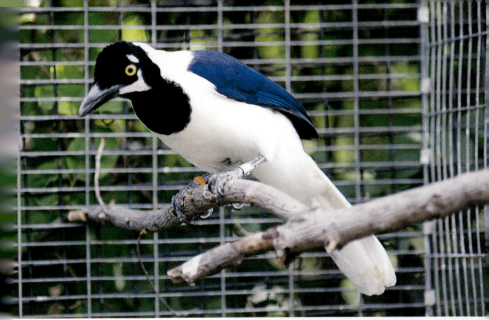

PASSERIFORMES

Crows, jays and magpies

Above: White-tailed jay,
Cyanocorax mystacalis.
Photo: Martin Vince

Right: Red-billed blue magpie,
Urocissa erythrorhyncha.
Photo: Bob Seibels

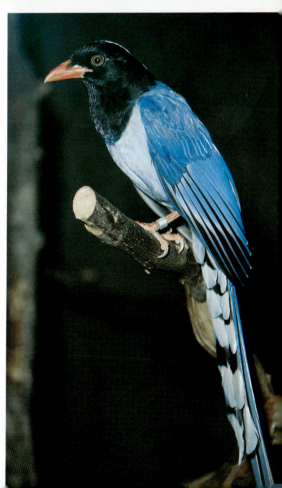

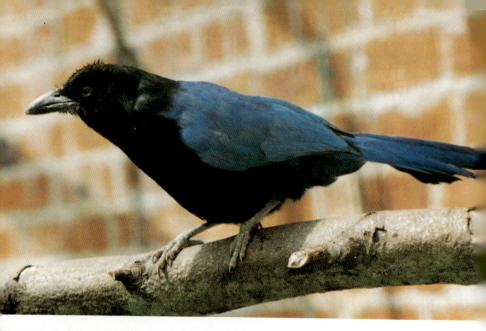

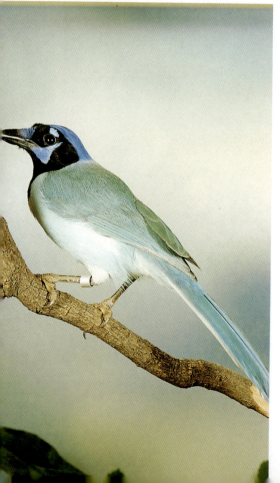

Above: San-blas jay, *Cissilopha sanblasiana*   Photo: Martin Vince

Left: Green jay, *Cyanocorax yncas*.
   Photo: Riverbanks Zoo and Garden

Tanagers

Right: Silver-beaked tanager (male), *Ramphocelus carbo*.

Below: Blue and yellow tanager (male), *Thraupis bonariensis*.
Photos: Martin Vince

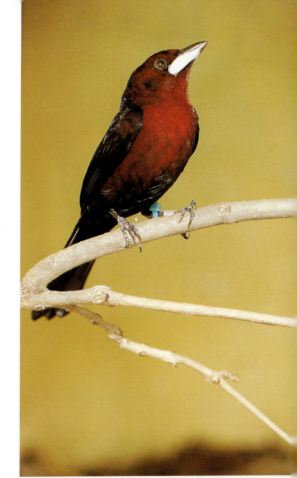

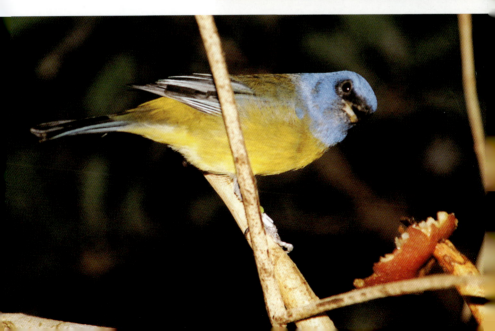

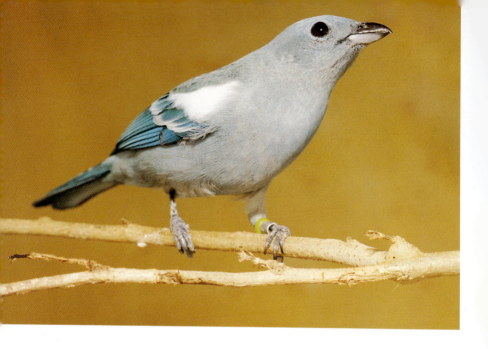

Above: Blue-gray tanager, *Thraupis episcopus*.

Below: Paradise tanager, *Tangara chilensis*.

Photos: Martin Vince

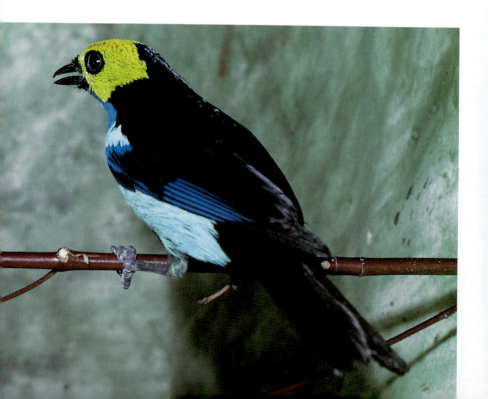

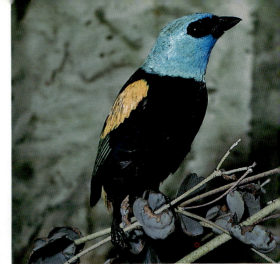

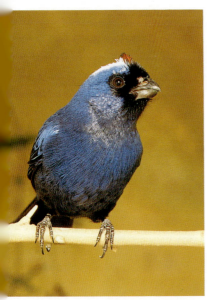

Above: Blue-necked tanager, *Tangara cyanicollis*.
Photo: Martin Vince

Left: Diademed tanager, *Stephanophorus diadematus*.
Photo: Martin Vince

Below: Bay-headed tanager, *Tangara gyrola*.
Photo: Bob Seibels

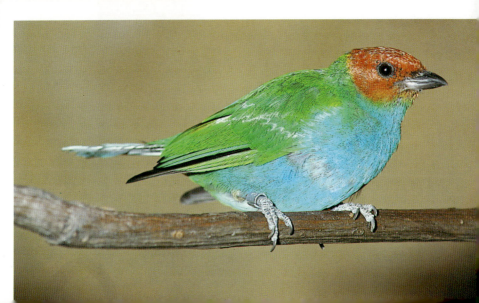

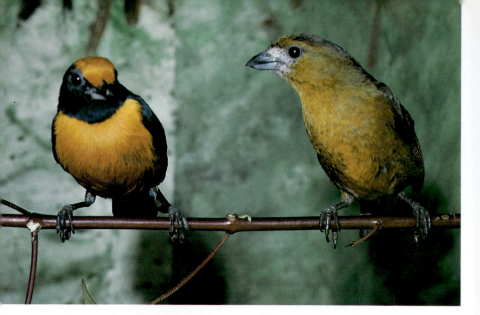

Euphonias and chlorophonias

Above: Pair of thick-billed euphonias, *Euphonia laniirostris*.

Photo: Martin Vince

Broadbills

Below: Lesser green broadbill (male), *Calyptomena viridis*.

Photo: Bob Seibels

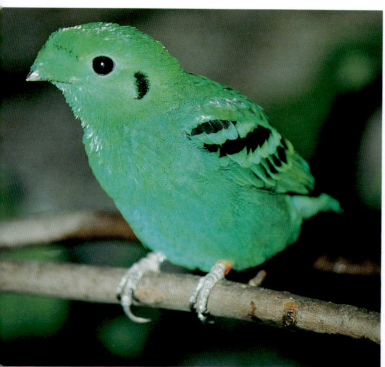

Opposite page:

Honeycreepers

Red-legged honeycreeper (male), *Cyanerpes cyaneus*.

Photo: Riverbanks Zoo and Garden

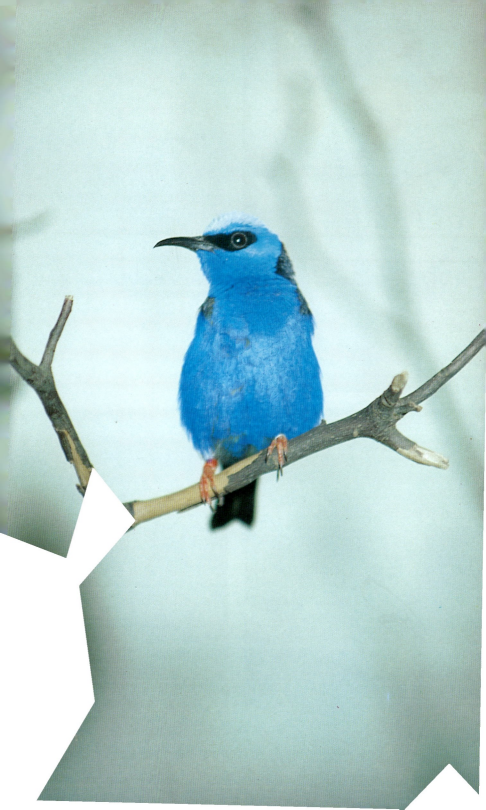

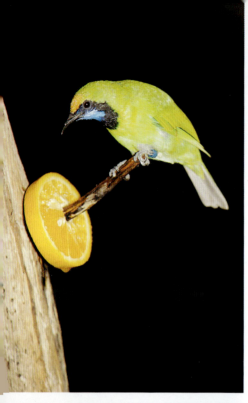

Chloropsis

Left: Golden-fronted chloropsis, *Chloropsis aurifrons.* Photos: Martin Vince

Lower left: Greater chloropsis (male), *Chloropsis sonnerati.*

Lower right: Greater chloropsis (female), *Chloropsis sonnerati.*

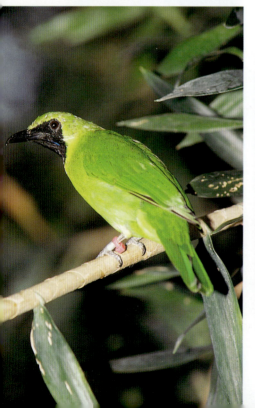

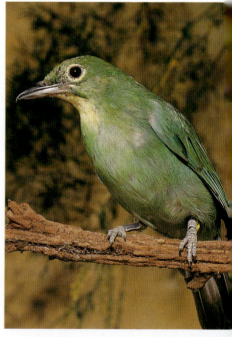

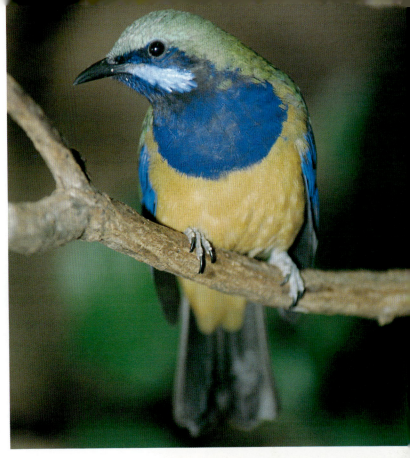

Above: Hardwicke's chloropsis (male), *Chloropsis hardwickei*.

Photo: Bob Seibels

Below: Hardwicke's chloropsis (female), *Chloropsis hardwickei*.

Photo: Barry Woodley

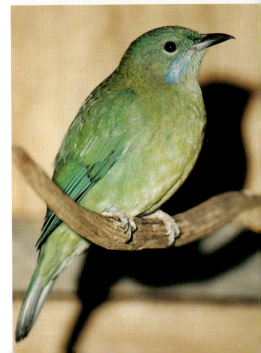

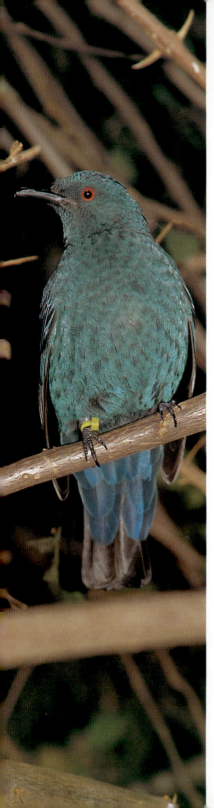
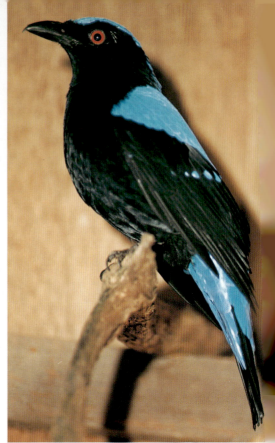

Fairy bluebirds

Above: Asian fairy bluebird (male), *Irena puella*.
Photo: Barry Woodley

Left: Asian fairy bluebird (female), *Irena puella*.
Photo: Martin Vince

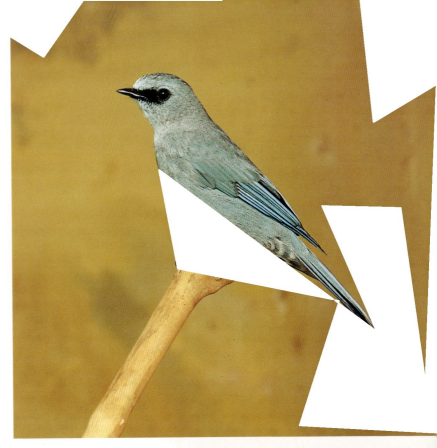

Old world flycatchers

Above: Verditer flycatcher (male), *Muscicapa thalassina*.
Photos: Martin Vince

Right: Greater niltava (male), *Niltava grandis*.

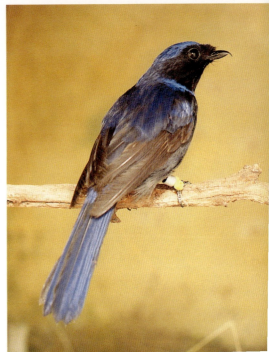

Pittas

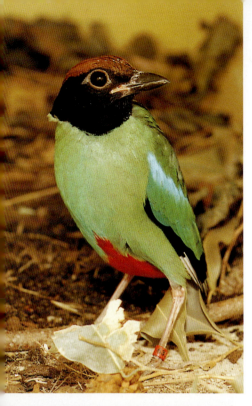

Left: Hooded pitta, *Pitta sordida*.
Photo: Martin Vince

Lower left: Banded pitta (female), *Pitta guajana*.
Photo: Bob Seibels

Bulbuls

Lower right: Red-vented bulbul, *Pycnonotus cafer*.
Photo: Martin Vince

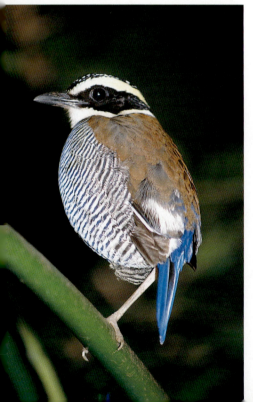

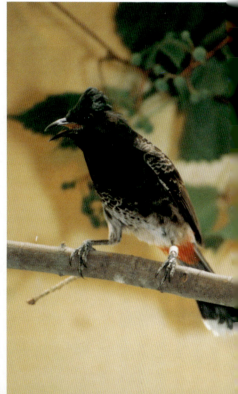

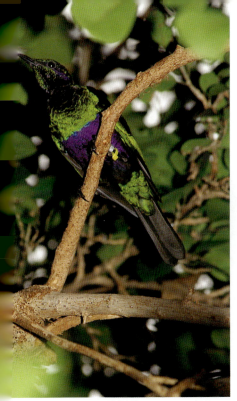
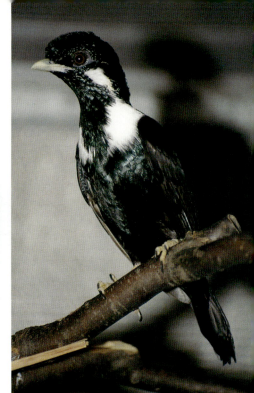

Starlings and mynahs

Upper left: Emerald glossy starling, *Lamprotornis iris*.   Photo: Martin Vince

Upper right: Sulawesi king starling, *Basilornis celebensis*.   Photo: Martin Vince

Right: Bali mynah, *Leucopsar rothschildi*.
  Photo: Riverbanks Zoo and Garden

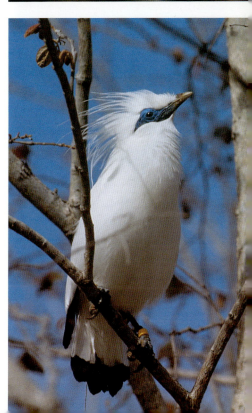

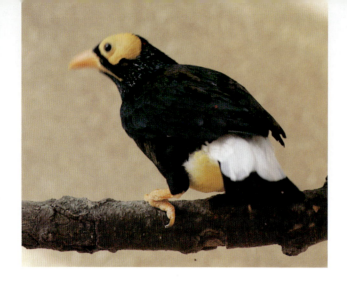

Above: Yellow-faced (Dumont's) mynah, *Mino dumontii*.   Photo: Martin Vince

Lower left: Asian pied starling, *Sturnus contra*.   Photo: Bob Seibels

Lower right: Golden-breasted mynah, *Mino anais*.   Photo: Bob Seibels

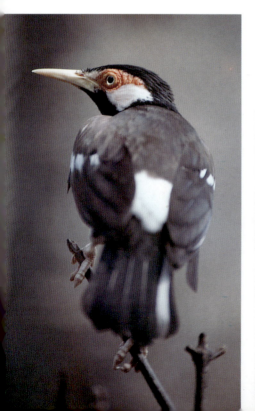

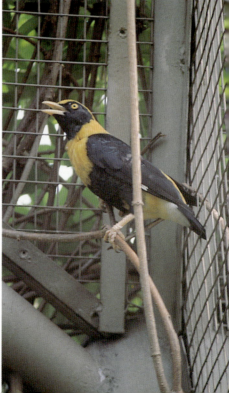

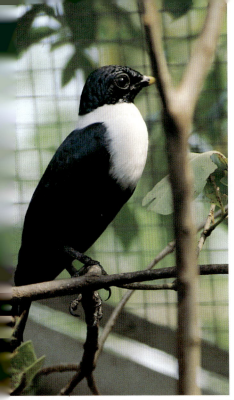
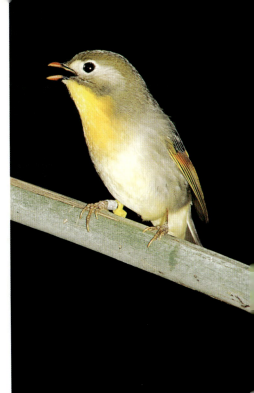

Upper left: White-collared mynah, *Acridotheres albocinctus*. Photo: Bob Seibels

Pekin robin and silver-eared mesia

Upper right: Pekin robin, *Leiothrix lutea*. Photo: Martin Vince
Below: Silver-eared mesia, *Leothrix argentauris*.

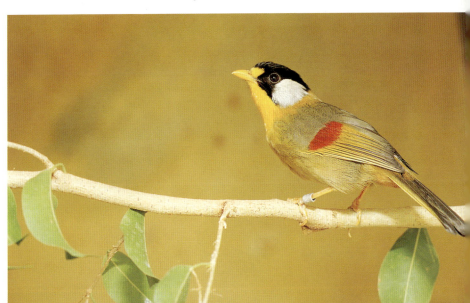

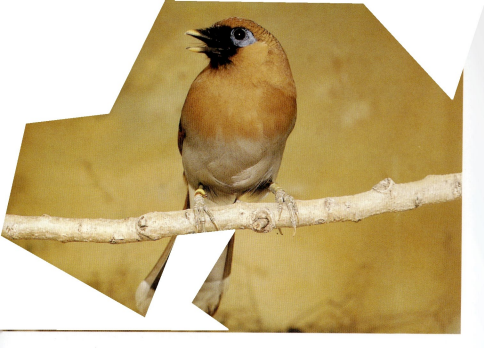

Laughing thrushes

Above: Rufous laughing thrush, *Garrulax poecilorhynchus*.

Below: Yellow-throated laughing thrush, *Garrulax galbanus*.

Photos: Martin Vince

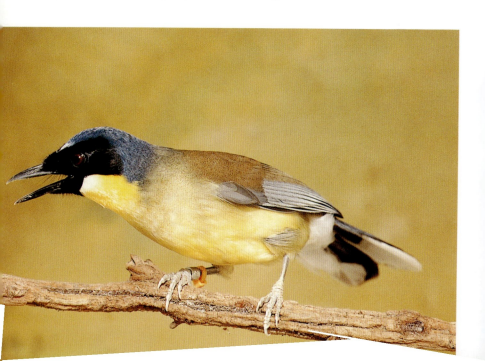

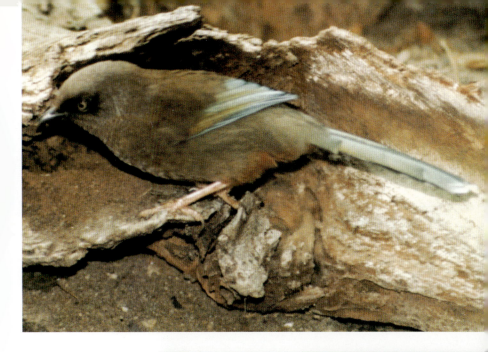

Above: Elliot's laughing thrush, *Garrulax elliotii*.
Photos: Martin Vince

Right: White-crested laughing thrush, *Garrulax leucolophus*.

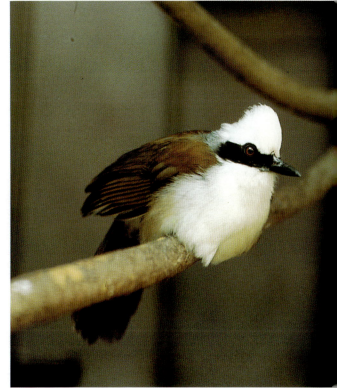

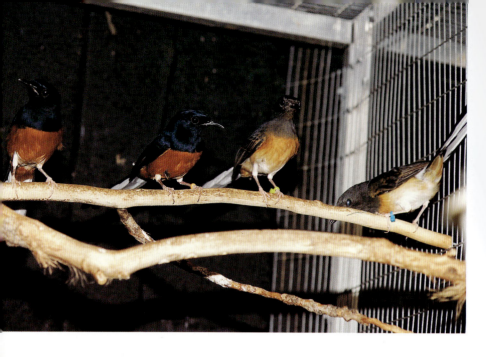

Shama and dhyal thrush

Above: Two male and two female white-rumped shama thrushes, *Copsychus malabaricus*—siblings aged 5 months. Adult shamas are naturally aggressive toward each other. These birds were each given their own aviary, soon after this photo was taken.

Photo: Martin Vince

Below: Dhyal thrush (male), *Copsychus saularis*.

Photo: Bob Seibels

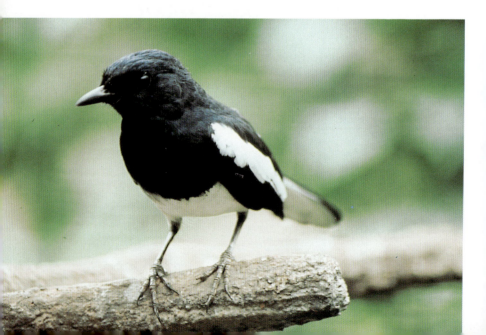

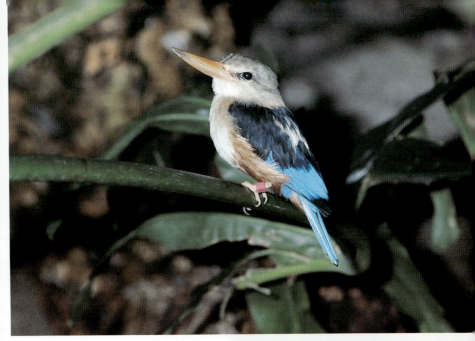

CORACIIFORMES

Kingfishers and kookaburras

Above: Gray-headed kingfisher, *Halcyon leucocephala*.
Photo: Riverbanks Zoo and Garden

Right: Guam kingfisher (male), *Halcyon cinnamomina cinnamomina*.
Photo: Bob Seibels

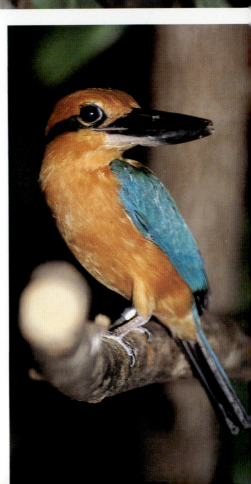

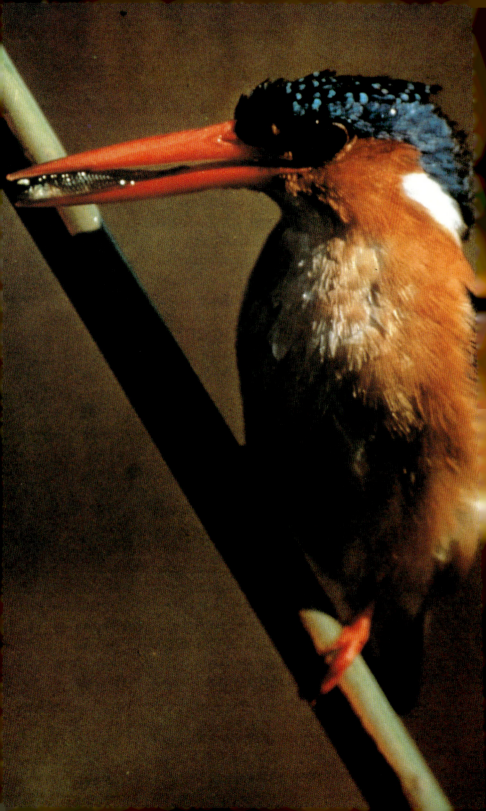

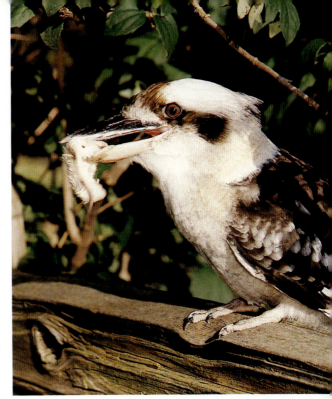

Opposite page: Malachite kingfisher, *Alcedo cristata*.
Photo: Riverbanks Zoo and Garden

Upper right: Laughing kookaburra, *Dacelo novaeguineae*.
Photo: Martin Vince

Lower right: White-collared kingfisher, *Halcyon chloris*.
Photo: Martin Vince

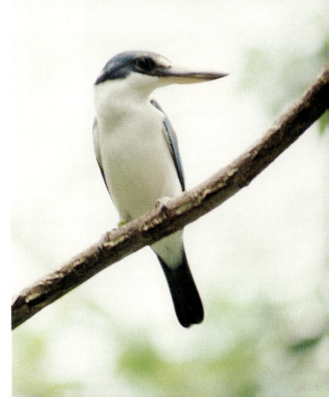

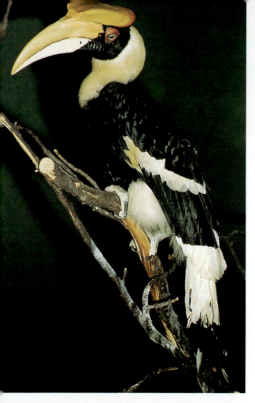
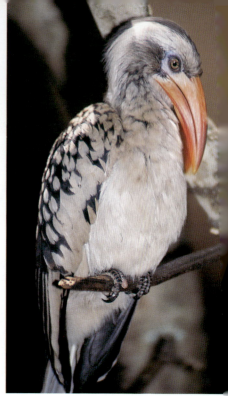
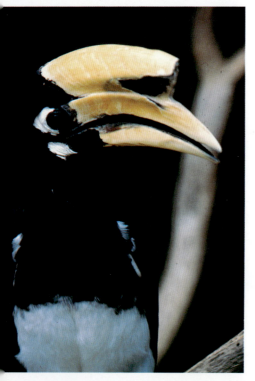

Hornbills

Upper left: Great Indian hornbill, *Buceros bicornis*.   Photos: Riverbanks Zoo and Garden

Upper right: Red-billed hornbill, *Tockus erythrorhynchus*.

Left: Northern pied hornbill, *Anthracoceros malabaricus*.

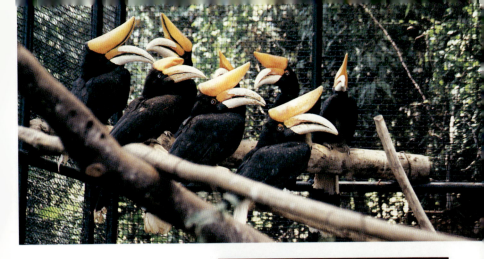

Top: Rhinoceros hornbills, *Buceros rhinoceros*. Photos: Bob Seibels

Middle: White-crowned hornbill (female), *Berenicornis comatus*.

Bottom: Blyth's hornbill (male), *Aceros plicatus subruficollis*.

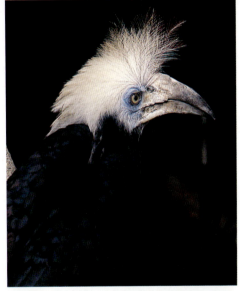

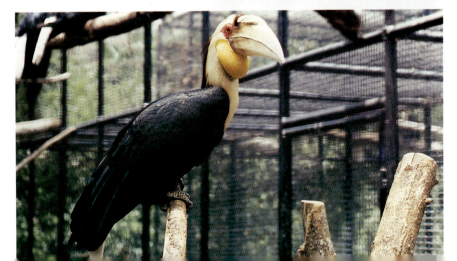

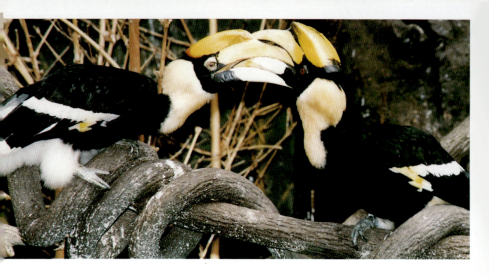

Above: A pair of great Indian hornbills, *Buceros bicornis*.   Photos: Martin Vince

Below: Jackson's hornbill (male), *Tockus jacksoni*.

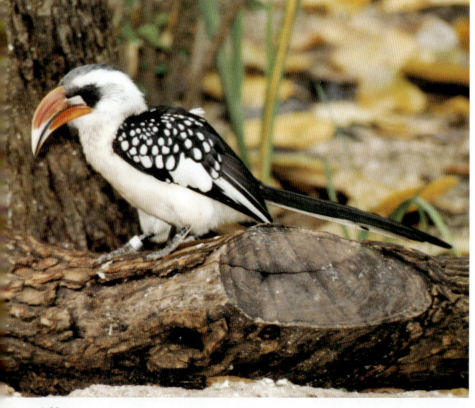

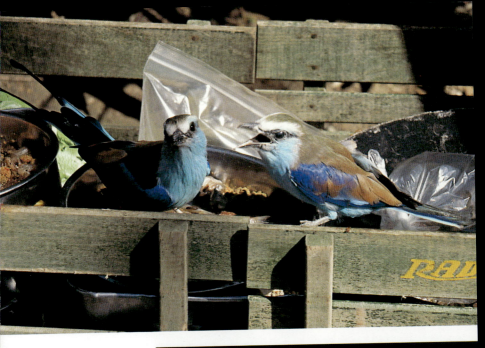

Rollers

Above: Racquet-tailed roller, *Coracias spatulata*.
Photo: David Hancock

Lower right:
Lilac-breasted roller, *Coracias caudata*.
Photo: Martin Vince

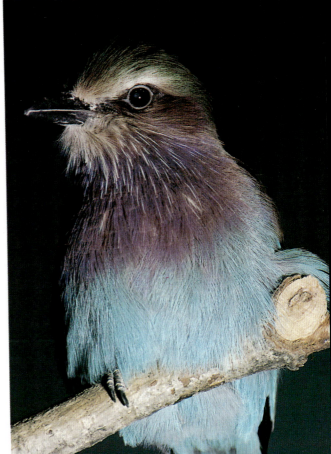

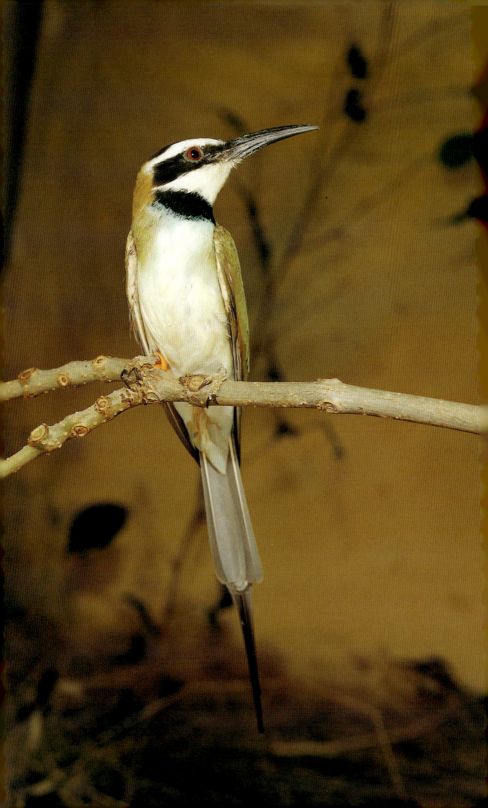

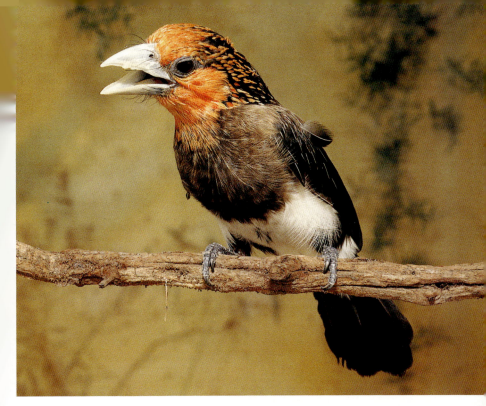

PICIFORMES

Barbets

Above: Brown-breasted barbet, *Lybius melanopterus*.   Photo: Martin Vince

Right: Levaillant's barbet, *Trachyphonus vaillantii*.
    Photo: Riverbanks Zoo and Garden

Bee eaters

Opposite page: White-throated bee eater, *Merops albicollis*.
    Photo: Martin Vince

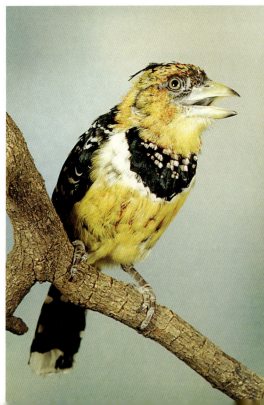

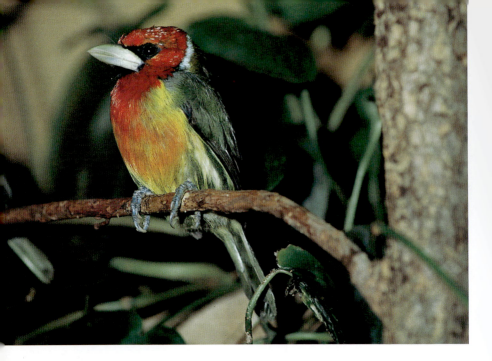

Above: Flame-headed barbet (male), *Eubucco bourcierii*.

Photos: Bob Seibels

Below: Fire-tufted barbet, *Psilopogon pyrolophus*.

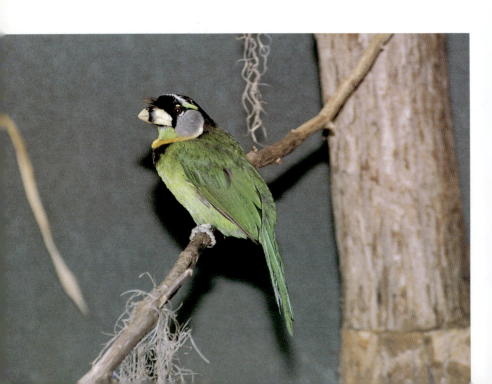

Toucans, toucanets and aracaris

Right: Green aracari, *Pteroglossus viridis*.
Photos: Martin Vince

Below:
Chestnut-mandibled toucan, *Ramphastos swainsonii*.

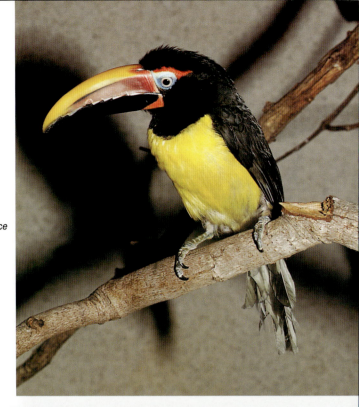

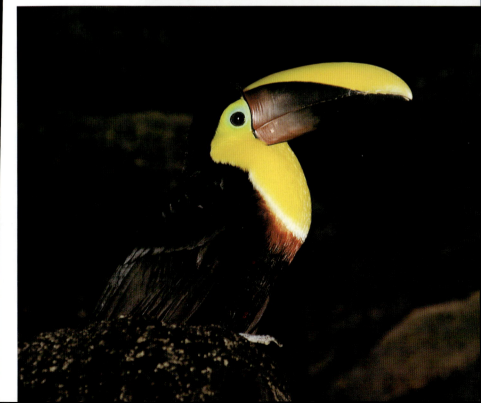

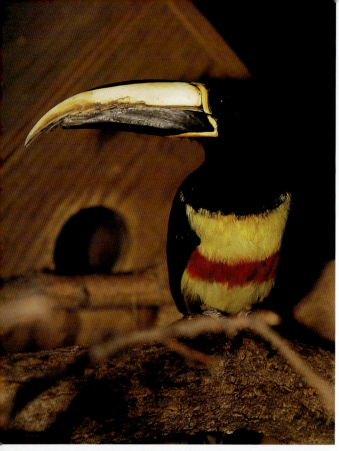

Left: Black-necked aracari, *Pteroglossus aracari*.
Photo: Martin Vince

Below: Saffron toucanet, *Baillonius bailloni*.
Photo: Riverbanks Zoo and Garden

Opposite page: Red-billed toucan, *Ramphastos tucanus*.
Photo: Bob Seibels

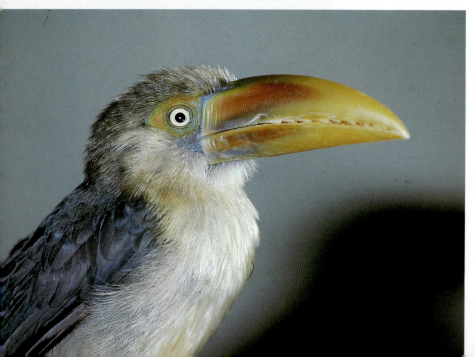

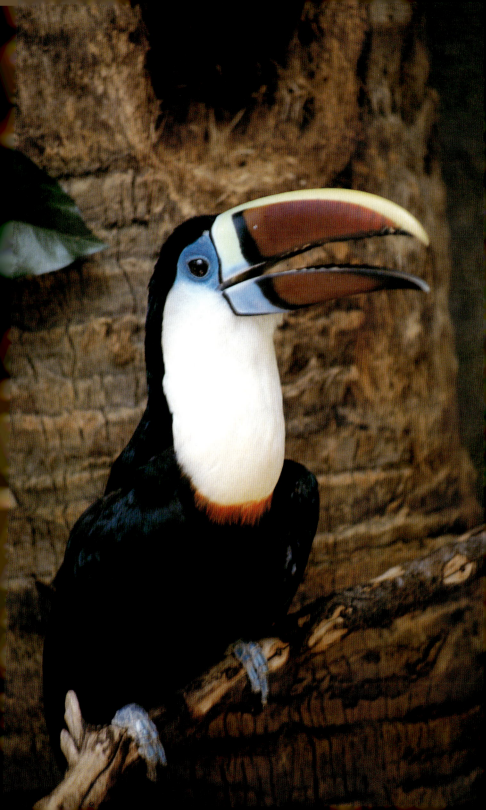

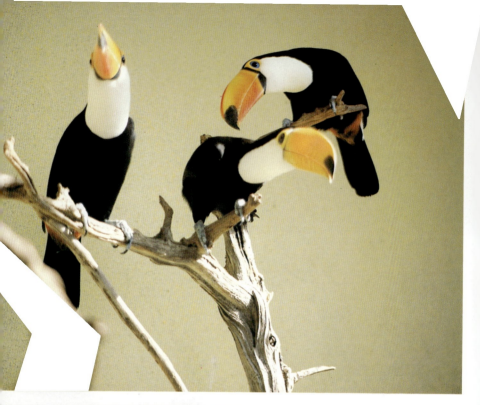

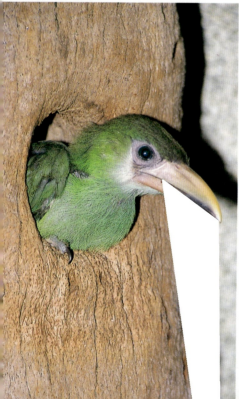

Above: Toco toucans, *Ramphastos toco* (adult pair with juvenile in middle).
Photo: Riverbanks Zoo and Garden

Left: Emerald toucanet (juvenile), *Aulacorhynchus prasinus*.
Photo: Riverbanks Zoo and Garden

APODIFORMES

Hummingbirds

Opposite page: Costa's hummingbird (male), *Calypte costae*.   *Photo: Martin Vince*

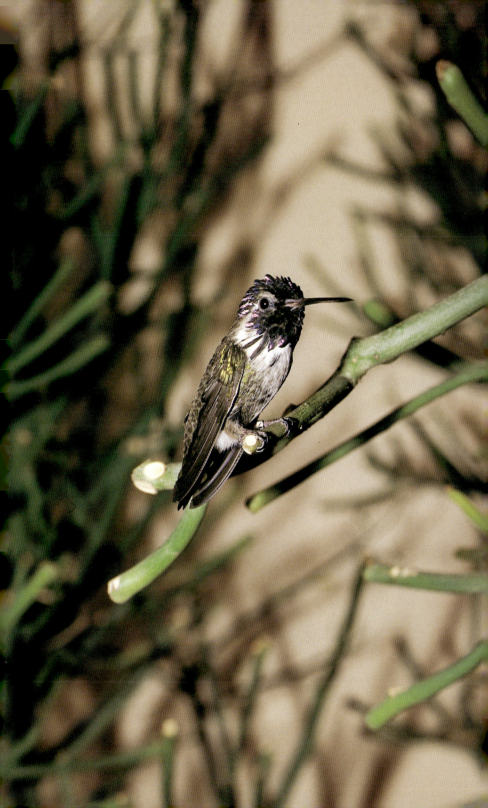

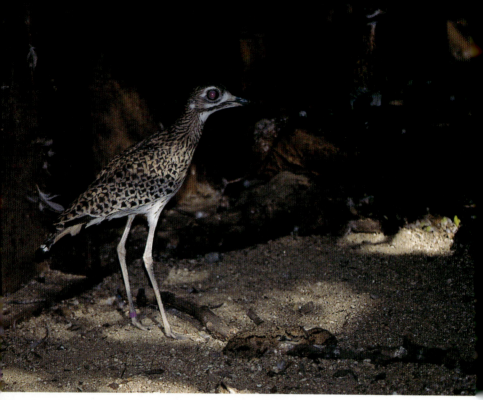

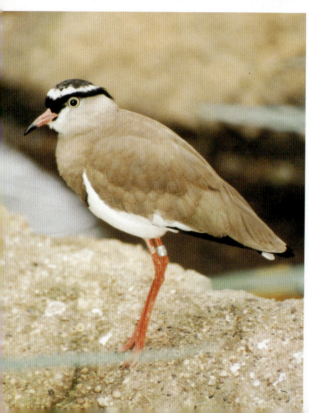

CHARADRIIFORMES

Lapwings and plovers

Above: Cape thick-knee, *Burhinus capensis*, with young.
  Photo: David and Laurel Hancock

Left: Crowned plover, *Vanellus coronatus*.
  Photo: Martin Vince

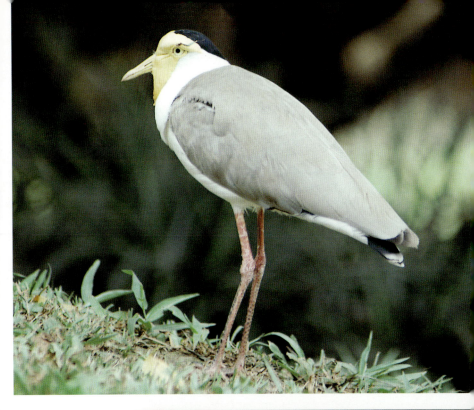

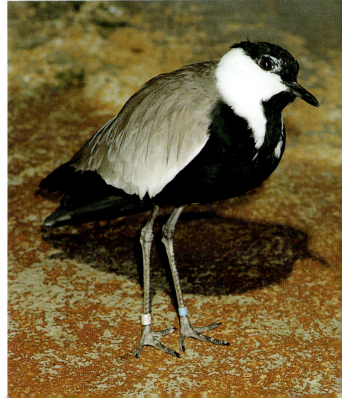

Above: Masked plover, *Vanellus miles*. Photo: Bob Seibels

Right: African spur-winged plover, *Vanellus spinosus*. Photo: Riverbanks Zoo and Garden

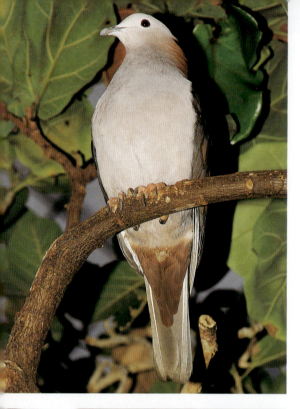

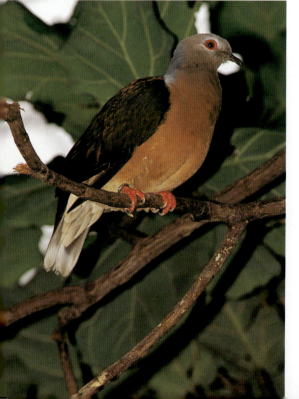

COLUMBIFORMES

Fruit doves and fruit pigeons

Upper left: Sulawesi green imperial pigeon, *Ducula aenea paulina*. Photos: Martin Vince

Lower left: Rufous-bellied imperial pigeon, *Ducula rufigaster*.

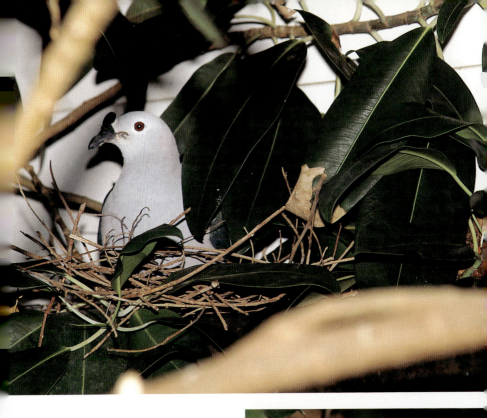

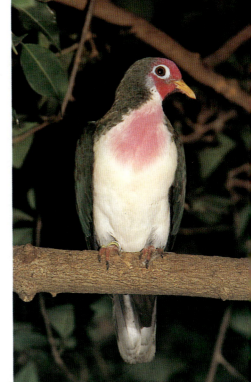

Above: Black-knobbed imperial pigeon (incubating), *Ducula myristicivora*.
Photos: Martin Vince

Right: Jambu fruit dove (male), *Ptilinopus jambu*.

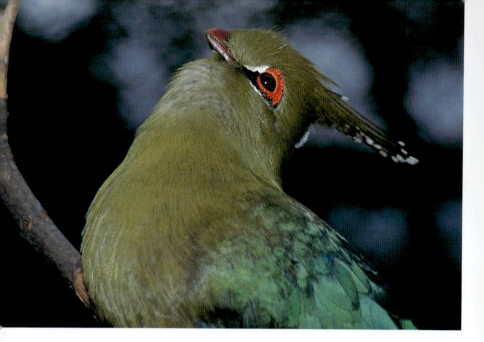

CUCULIFORMES

Touracos

Above: Livingstone's touraco, *Tauraco livingstonii*.

Photos: David and Laurel Hancock

Below: White-cheeked touraco, *Tauraco leucotis*.

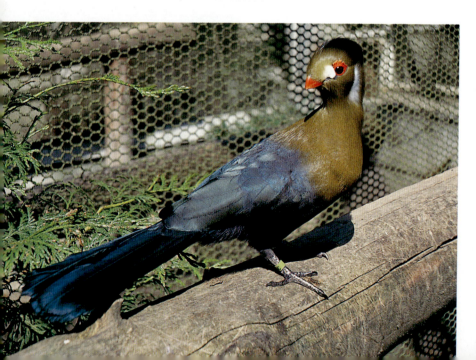

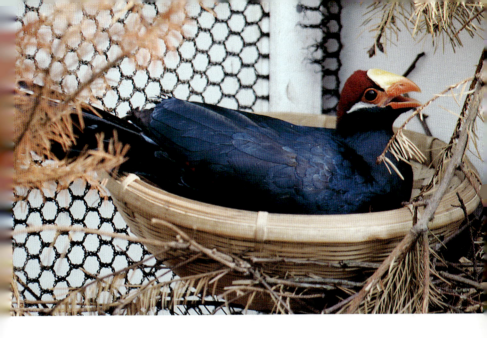

Above: Violaceous touraco, *Musophaga violacea*.

Photos: David and Laurel Hancock

Below: Red-crested touraco, *Tauraco erythrolophus*.

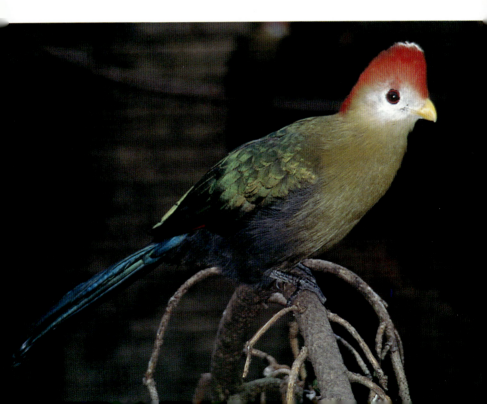

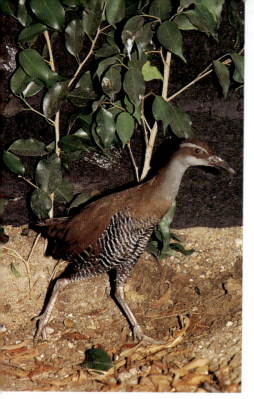
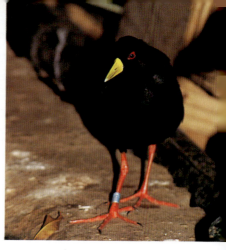

GRUIFORMES

Rails, crakes, coots and gallinules

Upper left: Guam rail, *Rallus owstoni*.

Photos: Martin Vince

Upper right: African black crake, *Porzana flavirostra*.

Below: Purple swamphen, *Porphyrio porphyrio*.

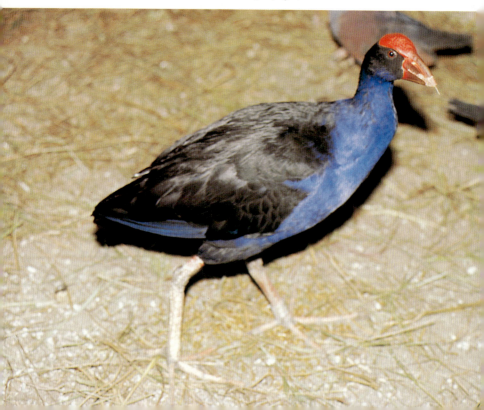

Tanagers

Order: Passeriformes
Family: Emberizidae
Subfamily: Thraupinae

Although a few tanagers are drab and unattractive, many are stunning and represent some of the most sought-after softbills. As well as the tanagers, Thraupinae embraces the *Dacnis*, flowerpiercers and the orangequit. It also includes the honeycreepers, and the euphonias and chlorophonias, which are aviculturally important groups in their own right, and described separately.

There are more than 240 members of Thraupinae, all of which have a purely New World distribution. Over 160 species are confined to South America, with 4 tanagers (genus *Piranga*) breeding in the United States and migrating to the tropics in the autumn. And many tanagers may undergo fairly local, seasonal migrations in response to food availability and rainfall cycles.

Over 60 percent of tanagers live in or near forests, and seem to have a distinct preference for areas that receive plenty of sunshine; and about 35 percent of species live in the Andes, where they are an important part of the local bird life. Almost all tanagers join in with mixed-species flocks, either straggling at the edge or helping to form the core around which others gather. Such flocks feed mostly in the forest canopy, on fruits, nectar and insects.

Size

Dacnis: 4–5 in. (10–13 cm).
Flowerpiercers: 4–6.5 in. (10–16 cm).
Orangequit: 5 in. (13 cm).
Most other common species: 6–7 in. (15–18 cm).

Compatibility (by genera)

Tangara species are usually safe with other birds, although pairs intent on breeding can become aggressive.

Thraupis species can also be aggressive when breeding, and generally tend to have a greater propensity for harassing others. It can be dangerous to keep them with smaller birds, except robust species such as the Pekin robin or silver-eared mesia.

Ramphocelus are similar to *Thraupis* tanagers, and can be even more spiteful when breeding—I recently saw a female silver-beaked tanager, *R. carbo*, chase a fairy bluebird into a window.

Anisognathus (mountain tanagers) are strong birds and should not be housed with smaller softbills.

Diet

Dacnis, flowerpiercers and the orangequit, diet F (see page 53) for nectivores. All other species, diet B (see page 51) for fruit-biased omnivores.

Management

Tangara species can be quite delicate when first imported, and need a diet that is soft and sweet. My preference is to mix equal parts of diced fruits and bread or sponge cake, that has been soaked in nectar and then squeezed dry. Once the birds have settled down and are feeding normally, they can be slowly converted to diet B. Most newly imported species from the other genera are relatively easy to acclimate, and should start eating diet B immediately.

When thoroughly acclimated, the following genera can be surprisingly hardy: *Thraupis*, *Ramphocelus* and *Anisognathus*. All of the species of these genera are capable of living outdoors year-round without heat. But they are not able to tolerate damp or drafty conditions, and must have a good quality, frost-free shelter. The most familiar examples of these hardy tanagers are the blue-gray, *Thraupis episcopus*; sayaca, *T. sayaca*; palm, *T. palmarum*; silver-beaked, *Ramphocelus carbo*; Brazilian, *R. bresilius* and the blue-winged mountain tanager, *Anisognathus flavinuchus*.

Tangara species are not usually so hardy, and should be given heated winter accommodation of at least 60°F (16°C).

To varying degrees, many tanagers eat the leaves of plants. This appears to satisfy some particular need they have, with *Ficus* trees often being favored. Damage can be considerable from just one pair of birds, but sometimes their attentions can be diverted if a piece of lettuce is given alongside the usual diet.

Breeding

Sexing: blue-gray tanager, monomorphic. Races vary greatly in their shade of blue; and juveniles may be difficult, or even impossible, to distinguish from the sayaca tanager.

Blue and yellow, dimorphic.

Silver-beaked, dimorphic.

Eggs: 2 or 3 in most tropical species; white to pale blue, usually with heavy, dark blotches.

Incubation: generally 12–14 days, and only by the female.

Most tanagers are monogamous and many live in pairs the year-round. One pair should therefore be given their own aviary. But in very large enclosures, 2 or 3 pairs may be kept together; and from such groups, potential breeding pairs tend to emerge more easily.

In the wild, the vast majority of tanagers build a cup-shaped nest in a bush or tree. In the aviary, artificial nest sites are very often accepted: half or fully open-fronted boxes, planted hanging baskets and cup-shaped wicker baskets should all be provided in secluded locations, and preferably within foliage.

For about the first week, the chicks are fed mostly live food. Provide plenty of mealworms and waxworms, which have been dusted with a multivitamin and mineral supplement to ensure proper nutrition.

After the chicks have fledged, they will continue to be fed by their parents for another 2 or 3 weeks. Once they are independent, they should be removed as soon as possible, since the adults may become extremely aggressive following a desire to nest again.

Euphonias and Chlorophonias

Order: Passeriformes
Family: Emberizidae
Subfamily: Thraupinae (Tanagers)

The approximately 27 euphonias and 5 chlorophonias are in fact members of the tanager group. But aviculturally they are best described separately to take proper account of their habits and requirements.

Euphonias and chlorophonias can only be found in the New World, and are mainly birds of the forest and forest edge, living in pairs and small flocks. Insects are eaten by both groups, and a few species are highly insectivorous. But for most others, fruits are the staple, and they are taken in the canopy and midheights of the forest.

Indeed all species are specially adapted for eating fruits, and the euphonias are well known for dispersing the seeds of parasitic mistletoe.

Size

All species, small and stocky.
Euphonias: 3.5–4.5 in. (9–11 cm).
Chlorophonias: 4–5.5 in. (10–14 cm).

Compatibility

They should all be relatively sociable in small groups or pairs, and usually live with similar-sized birds.

Diet

Diet B (see page 51) for fruit-biased omnivores.

Management

Most chlorophonias come from high altitudes and can be difficult to establish. They are not ideal for the beginner, although euphonias are much easier to establish and they tend to do well in aviaries.

Once they are established, euphonias and chlorophonias are quite hardy and certainly benefit from plenty of clean, fresh air. They seem to do best at 65°–70°F (18°–21°C) and can live outside year-round. Many species are capable of living through freezing weather without heat; but damp and wet conditions are always dangerous, and a warm, secure house that the birds can be shut into is recommended.

Breeding

Sexing: all species are dimorphic.

Euphonias: males are often a glossy blue, purple or yellow, while the females tend to be shades of dull olive. Females of certain species look so similar that in a mixed group, distinguishing between them is hard, if not impossible.

Chlorophonias: considerably greener than euphonias, with yellow or chestnut underparts. Females are similar to the males but not as vivid, with less yellow and generally a duller green.

Eggs: 3–5, usually pale with dark blotches.

Incubation: approximately 15 days, and only by the female.

Both sexes normally build the nest, which is domed, usually with a side entrance that may have a small overhang. The structure is built in the crotch of a tree, cavities in rock or wood, planted hanging baskets or among vines; and it is normally well hidden behind foliage. Nesting materials vary with species, but include: fine tendrils, fine twigs, mosses, leaves, fibers and grasses. Rarely, some euphonias in the wild use abandoned flycatcher nests.

In captivity, nests tend to be built in vegetation, although a half-open-fronted box and a wicker, cup-shaped basket are also worth trying. Both sexes rear the chicks, and feed them with regurgitated fruits and spiders. And therein lies the greatest difficulty of breeding euphonias and chlorophonias: many species will only accept live spiders when feeding very young chicks, and not just any spider will necessarily do. The birds will choose their favorite size and species, and that variety of spider will have to be supplied for at least the first few days.

Fledging times tend to be longer than for the other tanager species since the domed nests afford greater protection from predators. Chicks can remain in their nest for 3 weeks or more after hatching.

Honeycreepers

Order: Passeriformes
Family: Emberizidae
Subfamily: Thraupinae (Tanagers)

Like the euphonias and chlorophonias, these are part of the tanager group and purely neotropical. Honeycreepers have long, decurved bills and look quite different from the other tanagers. Indeed, it is only in recent decades that they have been incorporated into Thraupinae.

There are five honeycreeper species: the green, *Chlorophanes spiza*; short-billed, *Cyanerpes nitidus*; shining, *C. lucidus*; purple, *C. caeruleus;* and red-legged, *C. cyaneus*. They tend to inhabit the forest and forest edge of fairly dry regions, although the purple honeycreeper prefers more humid areas. Honeycreepers often travel in small groups, and sometimes feed with mixed-species flocks. Fruits and nectar are their main foods, with insects being gleaned from foliage and caught in midair.

Size

Short-billed: 3.5 in. (9 cm).
Other species: 4–5 in. (10–13 cm).

Compatibility

Pairs of *Cyanerpes* honeycreepers will usually live with similarly sized birds. But the more robust green honeycreeper can be slightly aggressive, and pairs should be given their own aviary.

Diet

Diet F (see page 53) for nectivores.

Management

I have imported the green, purple and red-legged honeycreepers; and using diet F, I have found that they are fairly easy to acclimate and establish. They will live in outdoor aviaries but should be shut into a warm house during cold or wintery weather.

Breeding

Sexing: all species dimorphic. The male red-legged honeycreeper has an eclipse plumage (out of breeding season) when he looks like the female; but he can always be distinguished by his red legs.

Eggs: nearly always 2, white or pale blue with brown spots.

Incubation: 12–13 days, solely by the female.

A pair should be given their own aviary with plenty of bushes and vegetation. The female alone builds a cup-shaped nest of dead leaves, rootlets, grasses and plant fibers; and cobwebs may be used to secure the rim of the nest to thin branches. In captivity, nests are also built in half-open-fronted nest boxes. This is to be encouraged since *Cyanerpes* nests are often so frail and thin-walled, that the eggs can be seen through them.

The chicks of *Cyanerpes* honeycreepers are fed by both parents, although the female does the bulk of the work.

The male and female green honeycreeper (genus *Chlorophanes*) can divide their labors to produce 2 broods in quick succession. The female feeds the chicks on her own for the first 5 or 6 days, while the male feeds the recently fledged birds from the previous clutch. Once they are independent, he returns to the female to help feed the second brood, which are now 5 or 6 days old.

Plenty of small live food is essential, including waxworms, mealworms, fruit flies and fly maggots. Nectar and soft fruits are also an important part of the rearing diet and should always be available. Once the young are independent they must be removed from the aviary, as their parents may nest again and become aggressive.

Pekin Robin and Silver-eared Mesia

Order: Passeriformes
Family: Timaliidae

Timaliidae is the large and diverse family of roughly 260 species of babblers, including laughing thrushes, liocichlas, yuhinas and barwings. Babblers are very lively birds that are constantly on the move, uttering a loud babbling sound as they go. The Pekin robin, *Leiothrix lutea*; and silver-eared mesia, *Leiothrix argentauris*; are probably the most well known of all babblers. For decades, they have been the staple of many bird importations and softbill collections, being colorful, small, hardy and undemanding.

Except when breeding, Pekin robins and mesias are highly gregarious, each living in groups of up to 30. And where their ranges overlap, they are frequently seen together, as they search the undergrowth for insects and fruits. They are often accompanied by other small babblers, and tend to keep within 15 ft. (4.5 m) of the ground. Indeed, they are as happy feeding on the ground as in the trees. Pekin robins and silver-eared mesias can be found in all types of jungle, but seem to prefer secondary growth, grass and scrub; and they live mainly in mountain and hill forests. Their range is great, with both species occurring in the Himalayas, Burma, Thailand, south and east China, Kampuchea, Vietnam and Laos. The mesia also lives in Malaysia and Sumatra. They are strictly resident, but like many birds of the Himalayas, descend to lower altitudes in winter.

Size

Pekin robin: 6 in. (15 cm).
Silver-eared mesia: 6.5 in. (16 cm).

Compatibility

Both species are safe with others. However, eggs of smaller birds may be eaten as breeding pairs can become aggressive with similar-sized and smaller birds.

Diet

Diet A (see page 51) for meat-biased omnivores. Color foods are also recommended to preserve the red, orange and yellow plumage, which otherwise fades after a period in captivity.

Management

These birds do not tolerate overcrowding, and will pluck each other if they are too closely confined. Newly imported birds can emerge from quarantine scruffy and plucked; but, if they are otherwise healthy, their plumage will recover at the next molt with no lasting damage. Severely plucked birds must be protected from the cold, so keep them at about 70°F (21°C) and only provide shallow bathing water until the missing feathers grow back—gently spraying them periodically with tepid water will help improve feather quality by encouraging preening. Once the plumage has recovered, deeper bathing water should be provided, since Pekin robins and mesias are enthusiastic bathers.

These are the easiest of softbills to keep, eating almost anything and thriving in most climates. Healthy specimens can live outdoors year-round, without heat, but should be shut into a frost-free house during severe weather.

Breeding

Sexing: Pekin robin males have a distinct song while females only utter call notes. In a group of mature birds, that all belong to the same race, have been exposed to the same levels of sunlight and fed the same diet, color differences between the sexes are fairly obvious. Males are generally brighter, especially the yellow and orange coloration of the throat, upper breast and wings. However, because of these variables, accurately sexing a single bird by its appearance is difficult.

Silver-eared mesia colors vary according to race, diet quality and exposure to sunlight. But in a group of the same race that has been kept similarly, color differences are obvious. The feathers on the rump and vent areas are red on the male and an orange-buff on the female. However, sexes are alike in the race from western Sumatra, *L. a. laurinae* (Delacour 1947).

Eggs: both species; 3 to 4 eggs, white to pale greenish blue with red-brown mottling, concentrated at the broad end.

Incubation: both species; male and female incubate for 14 days with a similar fledging period.

In a large, well-planted enclosure, a small group of mesias and Pekin robins live well together, and bring considerable life to the aviary. During the breeding season, pairs will break away from the main group and begin nest building. But if there is insufficient room for this, fighting will occur; so generally, a pair of *Leiothrix* should be given their own aviary. Alternatively, a pair can usually be housed with 1 or 2 females, year-round.

A cup-shaped nest is built in vegetation, normally within about 15 ft. (4.5 m) of the ground; and it is suspended either from a horizontal or vertical fork. Half-open-fronted nest boxes and cup-shaped nest baskets are also accepted. Some should be concealed behind vegetation, while others can be hung in more visible locations, since *Leiothrix* nests are not always well hidden. Nests vary in strength and composition, and include dry leaves, grasses, mosses, fine twigs, lichens and bamboo leaves.

In the wild, the breeding season stretches from about April to September. And both in the wild and in captivity, 2 broods can be produced each year. Chicks are reared by both parents and fed on live food such as small mealworms and waxworms for the first week or so, with the adult food included thereafter.

References

Delacour, J.:(1947) *Birds of Malaysia*. First edition. Macmillan.

Laughing Thrushes

Order: Passeriformes
Family: Timaliidae

There are about 48 species of laughing thrushes which make up the genus *Garrulax*. They are part of the large, Old World family of babblers, and nearly all of them travel in small, noisy flocks, with 1 bird whistling and another replying in a similar, but different song. With every bird in the group singing in such a way, laughing thrushes make themselves obvious to any passerby, although they are frequently hard to see among the vegetation.

Laughing thrushes are extremely active birds and often forage on the ground, turning leaves and debris for insects and fruits. They live in the dense evergreen and bamboo of India, the Himalayas, Burma, Thailand, China, Kampuchea, Vietnam, Laos and Borneo; some species live in forests and thickets at altitudes of up to 16,000 ft. (4,800 m).

Size

Large and robust birds: 9–14 in. (23–35 cm).

Compatibility

All of the laughing thrushes have the ability to kill smaller birds; and they enjoy eating eggs, nestlings, fledglings and any small animals they can catch. Even toward other laughing thrushes, a bonded pair is likely to be aggressive. Generally it is best to give a pair its own aviary.

However, some of the smaller species, such as the yellow-throated, *Garrulax galbanus*; red-tailed, *G. milnei*; and the red-winged, *G. formosus*, can live and breed with other equally robust birds. But the more pugnacious laughing thrushes, such as the white-crested, *G. leucolophus*; greater necklaced, *G. pectoralis;* and the hoami, *G. canorus*, are certainly better off in their own aviary.

Diet

Diet A (see page 51) for meat-biased omnivores.

Management

Like many other babblers, the laughing thrushes are particularly easy to acclimate and keep. They are hardy and readily accept an artificial diet, and bring considerable life to any aviary. All of them can live outside and do not necessarily need heat, but they should have a frost-free house as protection from severe weather.

Having said that, I have seen white-crested and greater necklaced laughing thrushes come to no harm, after having spent an entire winter roosting in snow-covered bushes.

Breeding

Sexing: monomorphic, although males may be slightly larger.

Eggs: 2–5, blue; some species plain, others with red-brown streaks and blotches.

Incubation: 13 or 14 days by both parents.

Laughing thrush nests are fairly well built and tend to be lodged in bushes and trees. They are cup-shaped and made of grasses, mosses, dead leaves, roots and creepers. In captivity, suitably dense vegetation will be utilized as well as half-open-fronted boxes and planted hanging baskets—the birds excavate a depression in the basket and fill it with the nest.

Once the chicks have hatched, live foods, such as mealworms, waxworms, pinkie mice and crickets, should be provided.

Sometimes, intelligent, semicarnivorous birds such as these, can become bored with the lack of foraging opportunities in the aviary; and they may turn on their chicks and eat them. Try to extend the birds' foraging time by throwing small amounts of live food into the aviary at regular intervals and by burying some live food in a tray of bran.

Once the chicks are independent remove them from the aviary as quickly as possible, to protect them from their potentially dangerous parents.

Fairy Bluebirds

Order: Passeriformes
Family: Irenidae

There are 2 species of fairy bluebird, the Asian or blue-backed, *Irena puella*, and black-mantled, *I. cyanogaster*. The 4 races of the black-mantled are found only on the Philippine islands of Luzon, Samar, Leyte, Basilan and Mindanao. They are shy and fairly uncommon, and unknown to aviculture. By contrast, the 6 races of the Asian fairy bluebird are quite common throughout their range, and have been avicultural favorites for several decades.

The Asian fairy bluebird inhabits the humid, tropical and subtropical regions of India, Burma, Thailand, Malaysia, Sumatra, Borneo, Java and the Philippine island of Palawan. It can be found in heavy jungle, and lives in pairs or small groups in the canopy of deciduous and evergreen forest. Fruits, berries and nectar form the bulk of the diet; and when trees are laden with fruit, many fairy bluebirds gather to feed alongside other fruit-eating birds. Indeed, the number of fairy bluebirds in a given location usually depends on the seasonal availability of fruits. And although this is not strictly a migratory species, it does travel locally in search of fruiting trees and bushes. It can be found at up to 5,000 ft. (1,500 m), but is more usually seen at lower elevations.

Size

Plumpish, thrush-like birds: 10 in. (25 cm).

Compatibility

Fairy bluebirds can be kept in pairs, and are normally safe in the company of other birds. But sometimes males become quarrelsome during the breeding season, and may represent a danger to smaller species.

Diet

Fruit-biased omnivore diet B (see page 51).

Management

Newly imported birds are relatively easy to acclimate, and usually eat the standard diet without any problems. But with finicky individuals, the diet can be made more enticing by adding extra live food and some bread softened in a sweet nectar solution.

Acclimated fairy bluebirds are easy to keep and can live outside year-round, with the protection of a frost-free and preferably heated house. Shelter from wintery weather is particularly important because fairy bluebirds have unusually small feet that are easily frostbitten; injuries from bumblefoot are also a possibility, and perches must be kept as clean as possible.

Breeding

Sexing: the Asian fairy bluebird, *Irena puella*, is dimorphic, and can be sexed at 5–6 months of age.

Black-mantled fairy bluebird, *I. cyanogaster*: *I. c. cyanogaster* (Luzon Island) monomorphic; *I. c. melanochlamys* (Basilan Island) monomorphic; *I. c. hoogstraali* (Mindanao Island) monomorphic; *I. c. ellae* (Leyte and Samar Islands) dimorphic (Delacour and Mayr 1947).

Eggs: 2 or 3 eggs; greenish cream with heavy blotching in purple or gray and brown.

Incubation: 13 days; incubation starts with the laying of the first egg and is done solely by the female.

The female Asian fairy bluebird builds the nest alone. It resembles the work of a thrush, and is made of thin twigs, grasses, animal hair and leaf fragments. In a well-planted aviary it can be built in the fork of a tree or in a bush; and half or almost fully open-fronted boxes are equally favored.

The chicks hatch a day apart. Both parents feed only live food for the first 3–4 days, with the standard adult diet included thereafter. Waxworms are the preferred rearing food, although mealworms will be taken just as keenly. Chick development is very fast: fledging occurs at about 12 days of age when the birds are fully feathered and surprisingly strong fliers. At about 4 weeks of age they are independent and should be removed from the aviary to make way for further breeding. Under ideal conditions, at least 3 broods a year can be raised.

References

Delacour, J. and Mayr, E.:(1947) *Birds of the Philippines*. First edition. Macmillan.

Chloropsis

Order: Passeriformes
Family: Irenidae

Alternatively known as leafbirds or fruitsuckers, *Chloropsis* are arboreal, often keeping to the treetops of heavy forest; but they sometimes descend to low bushes and even tall grass. Orchards and gardens are also frequented because they provide an abundance of the soft fruits and nectar-filled blooms that *Chloropsis* live on. Live food forms an important part of the diet, and *Chloropsis* spend a lot of time searching branches and acrobatically peering under leaves for insects or their eggs.

Chloropsis are fairly common in the wild, and come from India and Southeast Asia, including Sumatra, Java, Borneo and the Philippines. All 8 species are mostly green and have short, thick legs, and medium-sized wings and tails. They do not migrate although species in mountainous regions will descend to lower altitudes in cold weather. *Chloropsis* often live in pairs but can also be seen in flocks of 20 or more, especially at flowering and fruiting trees. They are beautiful singers and quite good mimics.

Size

Medium-sized birds: 7–8 in. (18–20 cm).

Compatibility

Chloropsis can be safely housed with other birds of equal or greater size, such as thrushes, tanagers, starlings and mousebirds. Smaller, robust species such as the Pekin robin, *Leiothrix lutea*, and Steere's liocichla, *Liocichla steerii*, also make suitable companions. Male *Chloropsis* can be aggressive toward females, and sometimes pairs will have to be broken up. But generally if a pair is released into a well-planted aviary together, the chances of success will be greatly increased as neither bird will have a territorial advantage.

Diet

Diet B (see page 51) for fruit-biased omnivores. Most *Chloropsis* have a great liking for waxworms which can be used to help bring them into breeding condition; but ration the food carefully, since waxworms are very high in fat. All *Chloropsis* need a separate dish of nectar in addition to their basic diet. For newly imported, sick or finicky birds, the food is more enticing if the nectar and basic diet are all mixed together in the same dish, making a sloshy food, similar to that enjoyed by lories.

Management

Chloropsis are very easy to cater to and eventually become quite tame; but be careful when handling them because their plumage is soft, and feathers can easily be damaged. Once acclimated, they are fairly hardy and will live outside year-round, provided they are shut into a heated house during cold nights or severe weather.

Chloropsis are well known for being aggressive toward their partners, except in particularly large, well-planted aviaries. Do not keep more than 1 pair of leafbirds in the same enclosure, otherwise fighting is likely.

Breeding

Sexing: most species are dimorphic. However, the 7 races of the golden-fronted leafbird, *Chloropsis aurifrons*, are monomorphic except *C. a. media* from Sumatra: the female has no black on the throat and the male has less orange on the forehead (Delacour 1947).

Eggs: 2–3 pinkish or white, with black or red-brown blotches.
Incubation: 13 or 14 days.

Ideally, a pair should be the sole occupants of a spacious, very well-planted aviary. A cup-shaped nest is built of fine grasses and roots in a tall bush, or fixed between twigs high up in a tree. Usually the nest is made in the most impenetrable and dense part of the foliage, and is impossible to easily see.

Chloropsis will also accept artificial nest sites. I recently saw a pair of greaters, *Chloropsis sonnerati,* use fine grasses and spider-plant leaves to begin nest building in a half-open-fronted box, and then in a thickly planted hanging basket. Eggs were not laid, although during nest building copulation did seem to take place: the male and female were perched 10 ft. (3 m) up, facing each other about 20 ft. (6 m) apart. She began fluttering her wings, and occasionally, briefly opened them while partially bowing and crouching toward the male. Simultaneously, he uttered a monotone, 10 part whistle which had a short break in the middle. All of this continued for 2 minutes and then the male flew to the female. He perched beside her and bounced over her, back and forth 3 times, before copulation which lasted about 5 seconds.

Soft-bodied insects, such as waxworms and molted mealworms, are vital as a rearing food. Nectar and soft fruits are always an important part of the *Chloropsis'* diet, and especially so when there are chicks in the nest. Once the young are independent, remove them from the aviary, because the adult male can become aggressive if he wishes to renest.

References

Delacour, J.:(1947) *Birds of Malaysia.* First edition. Macmillan.

White Eyes (Zosterops)

Order: Passeriformes
Family: Zosteropidae

White eyes are named for their prominent white eye ring; and most species belong to the genus *Zosterops* from which we get their alternative avicultural name. All of the white eyes display the distinctive white eye ring, except the yellow-spectacled, *Zosterops wallacei*; cinnamon, *Hypocryptadius cinnamomeus;* and olive-black eye, *Chlorocharis emilae*.

Zosterops are very widespread and quite common in mainland habitats. The approximately 85 species can be found in Africa and throughout Asia, including Indonesia, the Philippines, New Guinea, Australia and New Zealand. White eyes also live on many islands in the Pacific, including Hawaii where they have been introduced.

White eyes have brush-tipped tongues, short legs and rounded wings. The African species are mainly yellowish, while the Asian white eyes tend to be more green with gray underparts. But within this broad distinction they are all very similar with black, brown, white or gray markings. Though not colorful, white eyes are charming birds, that never fail to add considerable interest to the aviary.

Most species are active and lively, and live in small groups and flocks. They are purely arboreal and search for food in almost any area where there is sufficient tree growth; preference may be given to cultivated areas and gardens, where flowers and fruits can be found.

Size

Common avicultural species measure about 4.5 in. (11 cm): Indian or Oriental, *Zosterops palpebrosa*; chestnut-flanked, *Z. mayottensis*; and Japanese, *Z. japonica*. As a family, white eyes range in size from 3–5 in. (8–13 cm).

Compatibility

White eyes live well in single species groups and are unlikely to threaten other birds. However, during the breeding season most have the ability to be surprisingly pugnacious and may even injure smaller species.

Diet

Diet F (see page 53) for nectivores. With their decurved, pointed bills, white eyes are adept at catching small insects. Set up a fruit fly culture in the aviary and try to attract aphids with plants such as roses.

Management

The common white eyes are ideal for the aviculturist wishing to keep nectivores for the first time. They are fairly easy to acclimate and establish, being very inquisitive and willing to sample new foods. Established specimens are even easier to maintain, and are hardy enough to live outdoors year-round. Shelter from bad weather must be provided; and in temperate climates, frost-free and, preferably, heated accommodation is necessary. The provision of a night light is also important, allowing the birds to feed after dark and maintain good body condition during the coldest periods.

In the zoological environment, white eyes are one of the few birds that are able to live with crocodiles without being eaten.

Breeding

Sexing: white eyes are monomorphic, although mature males may be more brightly colored and marginally larger. Males also sing in the breeding season, whereas the females do not.

Eggs: 2–4, whitish or pale blue-green.

Incubation: 11 or 12 days.

When they are ready to breed, pairs will break away from the main group and defend their chosen nest site. Both sexes build a small, cup-shaped nest that is usually suspended between two horizontal twigs, or occasionally placed in an upright fork. The nest is built of grass-stems, plant down, animal hairs and cobwebs, high up in a tree or lower down in undergrowth and bushes.

Breeding success is more likely in a well-planted enclosure where the birds can build their own nest. But artificial sites, like cup-shaped, wicker baskets and half-open-fronted boxes, are also successful.

Both sexes incubate and feed the youngsters. The chicks fledge at about two weeks of age and continue to be fed by their parents for two to three more weeks. Small, soft-bodied insects are essential if the chicks are to survive; small waxworms, small mealworms (preferably molted) and ant pupae are all excellent food sources. Remove the youngsters once they are independent, because sometimes the adult male will chase the younger males. Two or 3 broods can be reared in a year, usually with a new nest built each time.

Sunbirds and Spiderhunters

Order: Passeriformes
Family: Nectariniidae

Nectariniidae comprises about 110 sunbirds and 10 spiderhunters. The sunbirds are widely distributed throughout Africa, the Middle East, southern China, India, and Southeast Asia including Indonesia and the Philippines. The olive-backed sunbird, *Nectarinia jugularis frenata*, can even be found in Australia. The spiderhunters have a far more restricted range and live only in Southeast Asia, particularly Malaysia.

These are the hummingbirds of the Old World, but they are not related; they cannot easily hover and certainly cannot fly backwards. However, they bear a resemblance in terms of their temperament and diet of nectar and small insects. The male sunbirds even have brilliant metallic plumage. The spiderhunters are less attractive, being mainly green and of a larger, heavier build, but they have a special charm and are excellent aviary birds. Most of the Nectariniidae have long decurved beaks for probing into flowers and long, hollow tongues for drinking nectar. Some of the sunbirds have shorter bills and reach the nectar by puncturing flowers at their base, in the manner of flowerpiercers and the bananaquit.

Sunbirds and spiderhunters are mainly birds of the tropics and inhabit almost all types of country. In Africa they live in moist savanna and forested areas, although some can be found in arid, desertlike environments; in Asia they frequent deciduous and evergreen forest, often preferring clearings and the forest edge. All are drawn to gardens and orchards, especially where bananas or plantains are grown. Some live in the mountainous regions of East Africa and in the Himalayas, Tibet, Nepal and south China, ascending up to 16,000 ft. (4,800 m) in the summer.

Size

Sunbirds are very small bodied with a total length that includes the tail of 3.5–6 in. (9–15 cm); up to 12 in. (30 cm) for some long-tailed males. Spiderhunters: 6–8.5 in. (15–21 cm).

Compatibility

On the whole, sunbirds are pugnacious by nature; and in the wild males defend favorite flowers, being especially hostile toward their own kind. They can be kept with other species, and those that do not compete for food, like small seed eaters, are probably the safest companions. Ideally a pair of sunbirds should be given their own aviary, since all species can become aggressive during the breeding season. Even pairs may not always live together, and particularly quarrelsome birds will have to be separated.

By contrast the spiderhunters are less aggressive and can be kept with docile, similar-sized birds. In fact, I once kept a pair of gray-breasted spiderhunters, *Arachnothera affinis,* with a pair of yellow-tufted malachite sunbirds, *Nectarinia famosa*, in a 10 ft. (3 m) square, planted aviary. Over a 2-year period none of the birds showed any aggression, even during the breeding season.

Diet

Diet E (see page 53) for sunbirds and spiderhunters. Red plumage fades after successive molts in captivity, and a color food is recommended.

Management

Newly imported sunbirds and spiderhunters can be infected with *Candida* and should be treated with Nystatin. (See Hummingbirds—management.)

Recently imported specimens tend to be delicate and need to be kept above 75°F (24°C). The nectar is also very important: a sudden change in the brand of nectar can cause a digestive disturbance and enteritis, which in a small bird can soon be fatal. Try to begin by using the same type of nectar as the previous owner, and if a change is made, it should be gradual. Do not actually mix the new nectar with the old, but offer 2 dishes of both types at the same time. Gradually reduce the unwanted nectar, until after about 10 days the bird is drinking only the new food. Using a probiotic preparation during the changeover can also help prevent illness.

Acclimated sunbirds and spiderhunters can live in a sheltered, outdoor aviary in the summer, but they need heated accommodation during cold weather. My preference is always to keep them at temperatures above 60°F (16°C), and provide a night light for continuous feeding.

Breeding

Sexing: sunbirds are generally dimorphic, with males exhibiting colorful plumage and sometimes longer tails. But the sexes of a handful of forest species are very similar; and at least the following sunbirds from East Africa are monomorphic: little green, *Nectarinia seimundi*; mouse-colored, *N. veroxii*; some races of the olive, *N. olivacea* and the Anchieta's, *Anthreptes anchietae*.

The males of some species have an eclipsed plumage, where they take on a duller, femalelike appearance outside the breeding season.

Spiderhunters have little or no difference between the sexes, and the males do not have an eclipsed plumage.

Eggs: 2 or 3; highly variable markings, but often pale colored with dark spots, streaks or scribblings.

Incubation: 13–15 days, solely by the female in the sunbirds; and by both sexes in the spiderhunters.

Sunbirds breed as monogamous pairs and should be the sole occupants of a thickly planted aviary. The nest is purse-shaped, usually with an elongated side entrance which often has a sort of porch. The spiderhunters build cup-shaped nests; and all species may use spider webs to help bind the nest or fix it to a substrate. Male sunbirds do not help in construction, but male spiderhunters will carry nesting material and may assist the female. Coconut fibers, grass, string, tissue paper, wool, animal hair and mosses can all be used. Nest building normally takes place in a tree or thick bush, although small platforms and finch or canary nest baskets are equally successful. These should be fixed in high, sheltered locations, including the aviary's house.

The male usually helps rear the young. Huge amounts of live food are required, such as fruit flies, aphids, fly maggots, and tiny waxworms and mealworms. Some sunbirds are particularly hard to rear because the adults will only feed certain spiders to their chicks; and unfortunately there is no easy substitute for simply collecting the live food from your back yard. Sunbirds usually fledge at about 14 days of age and start feeding very soon after. They are fully independent at about 4 weeks of age. At this point it is best to remove them, otherwise the parents are likely to become aggressive.

Shama and Dhyal Thrushes

Order: Passeriformes
Family: Turdidae

Turdidae is a large and almost worldwide family of roughly 330 species, that includes robins, chats, wheatears, redstarts, forktails and thrushes. But by far the most familiar members of this family are the common or white-rumped shama, *Copsychus malabaricus*, and its close relative, the dhyal thrush or magpie robin, *Copsychus saularis*. They are very similar birds, and share charming personalities and relatively straightforward requirements.

Shamas live in bamboo and evergreen jungle. They are fairly shy, and more often heard than seen, uttering their beautiful song and practicing a surprising capacity for mimicry. They feed very much on the ground, eating insects and occasionally fallen fruits, although they cannot be considered terrestrial and will comfortably fly high up into the trees when disturbed. The dhyal thrush has similar habits, although it is less shy, being a familiar visitor to gardens and a denizen of more open country.

The shama and dhyal thrush each comprise eighteen races that range from India, eastward to Burma, Thailand, Malaysia, Kampuchea, Vietnam, Laos, south and east China, Indonesia and Borneo. Dhyals can also be found in the Philippines.

Size

Dhyal thrush: 8.5 in. (21 cm).
Shama: Male about 11 in. (28 cm); female about 8.5 in. (21 cm).
In both species, tail lengths vary with race, age and sex.

Compatibility

Shamas and dhyals are normally safe with other birds. However, during the breeding season, males (especially shamas) can be extremely aggressive and are able to kill much bigger birds. As a result, a pair should be given their own well-planted aviary, although even this can be difficult.

Like many members of Turdidae, these are solitary birds; and whether a pair can live together depends upon their individual personalities, the size of the enclosure and the amount of vegetation and available hiding places. Many specimens are highly pugnacious and likely to kill their partner, while others are fine. When forming new pairs, try to acquire birds that are only a few months old, so that they can settle down and mature together. Generally, several shamas or dhyals can be kept in single species groups up to the age of about five months. But do not mix the species at any age, since fighting will quickly ensue.

Diet

Diet G (see page 53) for standard insectivores.

Management

Nowadays, most young shamas are captive bred and therefore easy to handle. But shamas, and particularly dhyals, are still imported and must be acclimated carefully if they are to thrive. Extra live food and very finely chopped, hard-boiled egg will stimulate feeding. And within 10 days of the birds' importation, the powdered softbill pellets will be eaten and the acclimation process will be well underway. But most important of all, these pugnacious birds should be quarantined in separate cages, preferably with visual barriers between each one.

Once acclimated, shamas and dhyals are quite hardy and are capable of living outdoors year-round without heat. But my preference is to provide at least some heat, and to shut them into their house during cold winters or severe weather.

Breeding

Sexing: shades vary appreciably between the races, but both species are dimorphic.

In shama, where the male is jet black and a rich chestnut, the female is slate gray and pale brown. Her tail is also shorter.

In dhyal thrush, where the male is glossy black and bright white, the female is dark brown and dark gray.

Eggs: both species; 4 or 5 eggs, dull green with brown-red mottling.

Incubation: in both species only the female incubates for 13 or 14 days.

Unless the pair have been living together successfully for some time, they will have to be introduced carefully. Keep them in adjacent aviaries, so they can see each other and remain in close contact. Hopefully, you can judge from their reactions and vocalizations, when they might be ready to breed. Introduce the male to the female's aviary by using a trap cage or preferably a connecting door, to reduce stress. The aviary should be as large and well planted as possible, offering plenty of natural and artificial nest sites.

In the wild, shamas tend to build their cup-shaped nests in vegetation, especially bamboo, while dhyals make use of tree holes, banks, walls and the roofs of houses. But in captivity both species use nest boxes with either a round entrance hole or a half-open front; and some specimens also accept cup-shaped baskets. In both species, the male and female usually build the nest and rear the young together. But fighting can break out at any time during the breeding process, and occasionally the male may have to be removed from the aviary—if necessary the female can easily raise the young on her own.

Plenty of mealworms and waxworms must be supplied as a rearing food. The chicks fledge at 13 or 14 days. In my experience (with 16 chicks last year) shamas are easy to sex at 3 to 4 months of age, looking like the adults, but with slightly shorter tails.

Pittas

Order: Passeriformes
Family: Pittidae

Pittas resemble thrushes in appearance, and have alternatively been called jewel thrushes, since some species are stunningly beautiful. Their bodies are stocky with short tails, long strong legs and broad, rounded wings; although they are not really designed for long flights, 8 species are migratory and travel long distances at night. All pittas are terrestrial, running and hopping with great speed, occasionally flying or freezing still, to take a discrete look back at their assailant. Pittas are extremely hard to see in the wild since they frequently take shelter in almost impenetrable vegetation, often being quite nervous and shy. Even with their sometimes brilliant coloring, they do not stand out in the half-light of the forest floor, and some birds are equally hard to see as they perch at the tops of tall trees.

The roughly 29 species are found in India and Southeast Asia, including Indonesia, Borneo, the Philippines, Japan and many South Pacific islands. Three species can also be seen in Australia and 2 more in Africa. Pittas live in various habitats, such as deciduous forest, scrub jungle or evergreen vegetation; and sometimes birds may venture into large gardens and comparatively open country. They are substantially or completely insectivorous and tend to be fairly territorial, with individuals usually only coming together to breed. Remarkably, pittas are thought to have a highly developed sense of smell, which they use to locate live foods, such as worms, that live beneath the surface.

Size

Plump, thrush-like bodies: 7–11 in. (18–28 cm).

Compatibility

Pittas are usually safe with other softbill species, and in largish enclosures will even live with similarly sized terrestrial birds, like crakes. But with other pittas they are often very aggressive, except during the breeding season when a pair may be kept together—even this is extremely uncertain and will depend on the compatibility of the individual birds.

Diet

Diet G (see page 53) for standard insectivores. Larger species also eat the occasional small mouse. In the wild, some pittas may eat fruit; but in captivity, fruits are not an important food and none of the species I have ever kept seemed to eat it. These species include: banded, *Pitta guajana*; giant, *P. caerulea*; Gurney's, *P. gurneyi*; hooded, *P. sordida*; or blue-winged (Bengal), *P. brachyura*.

Management

In my experience (with the banded, blue-winged and hooded), newly imported pittas are not difficult to acclimate and take quite easily to diet G. But if problems are encountered, diet H (see page 54) (for difficult insectivores) can be used in conjunction with the "meating-off" techniques.

Being terrestrial, pittas have fairly delicate feet which are quickly damaged by hard surfaces such as concrete or dirt. To avoid such foot ailments as "bumblefoot," it is therefore essential that pittas are provided with a soft floor covering of peat moss and leaves. This should be kept moist at all times to prevent dust from causing eye and respiratory problems. Although largely terrestrial, pittas will perch several feet above the ground, and should have at least one high perch for roosting; a rotting log will also provide a low perch for use during the day.

Breeding

Sexing: dimorphic: giant, banded and Gurney's
Monomorphic: blue-winged (Bengal) and hooded.
Eggs: usually 3–5, with an incubation of 15–17 days.

The key to success is persuading a pair of pittas to live together long enough to breed; and even if all appears to be going well, injury or death is always a possibility. The intended pair should be housed within sight of each other and preferably in adjacent aviaries prior to the introduction. Spend as much time as possible observing them. They should already be in peak condition, and if there appears to be little or no aggression, they can be introduced. A small amount of aggression and chasing is a fairly normal prelude to mating. However, if the female is not in full breeding condition, fighting and injury can occur. Constant observation is essential with most pairs.

Soon after copulation, both sexes start building a rough, globular or elliptical nest, which can be as big as a soccer ball. It is normally built on the ground or lodged in the low branches of a tree or bush, but nests may also be built as high as 30 ft. (9 m) up. Dried leaves and grasses are usually held together with strips of fiber, or twigs and roots; and the interior is lined with fine twigs, grasses and green leaves. An entrance hole is made on the side, often with a kind of platform beneath it.

Both sexes share rearing duties, feeding a variety of live food to the chicks. It is important to remove the youngsters as soon as they become independent, since the adults may quickly turn on them following a desire to renest. Indeed, aggression between the adults can sometimes flare up at this point if both birds are not ready to build another nest and breed again; and it may be necessary to separate the adults and pair them again soon after.

Old World Flycatchers

Order: Passeriformes
Family: Muscicapidae

Muscicapidae includes such familiar flycatchers as the verditer, *Muscicapa thalassina*; Japanese blue, *Cyanoptila cyanomelaena;* and all of the *Niltava* species. But throughout the world there are considerably more flycatchers from various families, such as the approximately 31 species of puffback flycatchers and wattle-eyes (family Platysteiridae) of mostly North Africa. These small softbills are rarely exported. They tend to be slightly delicate and difficult to acclimate. They should be protected from dampness and drafts, and maintained at least 75°F. The finest, most powdery insectivorous diet (G) is also essential.

By far the greatest concentration of flycatchers can be found in the New World. There are nearly 400 species of Tyrant flycatchers (family Tyrannidae), and it is amazing that most are unknown to aviculture. This is presumably due to a lack of enterprising exporters, rather than the birds' avicultural difficulty.

The Old World flycatchers live mainly on insects, and can be found in almost any wooded area, from mixed deciduous to open evergreen forest. Many species hawk insects from a conspicuous perch. Their bills are broad, flattish and bristled around the nostrils. There are also a great many species with much finer bills that search for food in foliage, while others will take prey from the ground.

Muscicapidae covers a tremendous range, with species in Africa, Europe and throughout Asia and Southeast Asia, including Indonesia and the Philippines; and some have even reached New Zealand and the Hawaiian islands. In tropical regions, most flycatchers are resident, but species that breed in Europe, avoid the cold winters by migrating to Africa, India and Southeast Asia.

Size

Small to medium sized: 4–8.5 in. (10–21 cm). The female paradise flycatchers are about 8 in. (20 cm); and due to their tails, the male birds measure an additional 9 in. (23 cm) in length.

Compatibility

Single specimens are usually docile and live with other birds as small as tits. Flycatchers' bodies are not especially robust and must be protected from overbearing species that may cause injury. A pair of flycatchers will very often live together year-round without any aggression, but may start fighting as the breeding season approaches; and problems are almost guaranteed if flycatcher pairs are mixed together.

Diet

Diet G (see page 53) for standard insectivores, made as fine and powdery as possible.

Management

Newly imported specimens are sometimes thin if they have not been eating properly during the importation process. In the short-term, extra live food is usually essential to prevent death. But after about 10 days the birds start eating the artificial food, provided the ingredients are ground up into a fine powder and moistened according to the diet G recipe. Eating the artificial food is vital for long-term health, since a diet of purely mealworms, waxworms and crickets, quickly leads to malnutrition and death. It is for such reasons that the specialist aviculturist has the most success with insectivores, which so easily come to grief in less-experienced hands.

A healthy, properly acclimated flycatcher or *Niltava* can be surprisingly hardy, coming, as many of them do, from high altitudes. I have seen several species perch outside in snow for long periods, suffering no ill effects; but on a wintery night, flycatchers should be shut into a heated house that is fitted with a night light to allow continuous feeding.

Breeding

Sexing: all Old World species commonly kept in aviculture are dimorphic.

Eggs: 3–5 for the common, avicultural species
Incubation: 12–14 days for the common species

I have never had any trouble keeping *Niltava* or flycatcher pairs together; but if the male comes into breeding condition before the female, quarreling or fighting can be expected and they may have to be separated. Keep the birds in view of each other and preferably in adjacent aviaries. An increase in vocalizations, and the birds' general demeanor should indicate the readiness to breed, and if both birds are in perfect condition they can be re-paired. Before the introduction, add more plants and nest sites to the aviary. This will provide plenty of hiding places, and create the secluded effect that is conducive to breeding. As with most softbills, breeding success is far more likely if the pair are given their own aviary.

Flycatchers are often found in relatively open country, but retreat to denser forests to breed. Nests are usually a small cup of mosses, lichens, dry leaves and grasses, lined with fine roots and animal hair. They can be built from 5–40 ft. (1.5–12 m) in a tree, lodged among branches, or in a hole or hollow found in rock work, banks or tree trunks. In captivity, a pair of flycatchers is far more likely to build a nest in a half-open-fronted box than foliage. Cup-shaped wicker baskets should also be offered, with all nest sites concealed behind plants.

The chicks will need a constant supply of live food, which must be as small as possible for the first few days. "Mini" maggots that are about 6 mm long can be fed directly to the birds; or the miniature flies they produce are even better. Put some maggots in a jar with small holes in the lid, and leave the jar in the aviary. Allow the maggots to metamorphose into flies; as they emerge through the holes, they will be picked off by the flycatchers. Flies alone are not a nutritious rearing food, and it is important to provide small waxworms and mealworms, and any ant pupae you have in the freezer or can collect. Dust all of the live foods with a multivitamin and mineral supplement. The chicks only take 2 to 3 weeks to fledge and are independent after a similar period.

Broadbills

Order: Passeriformes
Family: Eurylaimidae

There are 14 broadbill species. Four occur in Africa with the remainder found in the Himalayas and throughout Southeast Asia, including the Philippines, Borneo and Indonesia. They are stocky birds with a wide gape, large eyes, short legs and generally, elongated tails. Most, like the long-tailed broadbill, *Psarisomus dalhousiae*, are highly insectivorous and use their wide bills to catch insects on the wing, but may also take prey from the ground, including very small lizards and frogs. However, the 3 species that comprise the genus *Calyptomena* feed mainly on soft fruits and buds, and are therefore much easier to keep in captivity. This includes the lesser green broadbill, *C. viridis*, which has been an avicultural favorite since the beginning of this century.

Broadbills are often gregarious, living in small groups or flocks. Most can be found in dense evergreen or mixed deciduous forest; and while some may come into the open to feed, they will usually remain close to heavy vegetation.

Size

Small to medium: 5–11 in. (13–28 cm). Lesser green: 7.5 in. (19 cm); long-tailed 11 in. (28 cm).

Compatibility

Broadbills are docile with all other birds, but should be protected from over-bearing species that may monopolize the food and almost certainly prevent breeding. In large aviaries, groups of broadbills should live amicably together: I have kept 5 lesser greens (3 females and 2 males) in an aviary 20 ft. x 30 ft. x 8 ft. high, without any problems. And 2 pairs of long-tailed broadbills were kept in a similarly sized aviary with equal success. In each case the broadbills were housed with birds such as fruit doves, liocichlas, Pekin robins, ground thrushes and *Chloropsis*.

Diet

Lesser green broadbill: diet B (see page 51) for fruit-biased omnivores. Newly purchased or imported birds can be finicky and should receive a lot of clearly visible berries and diced fruits. Once the bird is feeding normally, gradually decrease the fruit content until the diet B recipe is achieved.

Live food, and especially avocados, can be used to help bring broadbills into breeding condition. However, outside of the breeding season, my preference is to completely avoid avocados because they are potentially dangerous. (See nutrition—vitamin E.)

Long-tailed broadbill: diet H (see page 54) for newly imported birds; diet G for established specimens.

Management

Coming, as they do, from dense forest, it is not surprising that broadbills can be nervous birds and may stress easily. Provide them with foliage or something they can hide behind, especially if they are already in a stressful environment such as a small cage. A large, well-planted aviary or tropical house provides the ideal broadbill accommodation, and since they tend to nest near water, a small pool or stream is worthwhile. Even when acclimated, the lesser green broadbill cannot endure cold or drafts, and should be given heat during the winter of at least 55°F (13°C). The long-tailed broadbill is normally more hardy, but still needs warmth during wintery weather.

Breeding

Sexing: lesser green broadbill, dimorphic. Long-tailed broadbill, monomorphic.

Eggs: lesser green: 2 eggs; white or pinkish, either plain or with reddish brown blotches.

Long-tailed: 5 or 6 eggs; white or pinkish with reddish brown blotches.

Incubation: lesser green, 17 days.

Keeping a small group of broadbills in a large, planted aviary will provide the best chances of breeding, especially for the long-tailed broadbill, which has been seen in flocks of 30 in the wild. Once a pair has been formed, it breaks away from the main group to build a nest and breed. It has been suggested that male lesser green broadbills perform their courtship displays communally, in specific areas (or leks), and that at least this broadbill species may be polygynous. However, research is still required and the lesser green remains something of a mystery.

Broadbills' nests are well camouflaged, looking like a mass of debris hanging from an exposed branch, often over water. They are further disguised by lichens, pieces of bark and cobwebs, and fibers hanging roughly from the base. In the middle is a chamber, lined with fibers and leaves, and access is often gained via a hole on the side which may be canopied.

In captivity, if a pair is keen to breed, but is merely unable to build a cohesive structure, large teardrop shapes can be made from wire mesh, natural fiber doormats or palm leaves. They should be hung from a high branch and thickly lined with materials such as grasses, hay, straw, leaves, mosses and plant fibers.

When broadbills are feeding chicks, their need for live food and soft fruits, sometimes avocado, increases. Provide plenty of molted mealworms and waxworms, along with bread or cake soaked in a nectar solution. See diet F, for nectivores. Soak the bread and squeeze it until fairly dry, and sprinkle it on top of the diet.

Bulbuls

Order: Passeriformes
Family: Pycnonotidae

The bulbuls, greenbuls and brown bulbuls form the bulk of this Old World, and mainly tropical, family of about 120 species. They can be found in Africa, and from the Middle East to Japan, Southeast Asia, Indonesia and the Philippines. Most species live in the equatorial rainforests of Africa and similar habitats in Southeast Asia. Although nearly all of the bulbuls known to aviculture come from Southeast Asia, the greatest number of species are found in Africa.

Bulbuls are fairly noisy and easy to detect, and live mostly in pairs or small groups, congregating in far greater numbers to feed at fruiting trees. Bulbuls often keep to the higher reaches of the forest and woodland, but sometimes join together in lower trees, and boldly enter orchards and gardens. The red-whiskered bulbul, *Pycnonotus jocosus*, is the best example of this, feeding on cultivated fruits and benefitting greatly from human occupation.

Nearly all species are dully colored in olives and browns, with paler underparts; but many are crested and have attractive red or yellow plumage about the vent.

Size

Medium-sized birds: 5–9 in. (13–23 cm).

Compatibility

Many bulbuls are docile, and can usually be housed with other bulbuls and similar-sized birds. However, some specimens are aggressive, especially males during the breeding season. More than one pair of bulbuls may breed in the same aviary, but territories will be defended and a careful watch must be maintained. Ideally each pair should be given their own aviary, if at all possible.

Diet

Diet B (see page 51) for fruit-biased omnivores. Bulbuls are very easy to feed and will eat almost anything. Two or 3 mealworms or waxworms can be given each day, but they are very fattening and not essential in a maintenance diet.

Management

The commonly available bulbuls are ideal birds for the beginner: red-whiskered, *Pycnonotus jocosus*; red-vented, *Pycnonotus cafer*; yellow-vented, *Pycnonotus goiavier*; and the white-cheeked, *Pycnonotus leucogenys*. They are all undemanding birds, quite attractive and melodious; they do not need heat and are hardy enough to stay outside year-round provided they have the protection of a frost-free shelter.

Breeding

Sexing: monomorphic.
Eggs: 2–5, purplish pink, often speckled in reddish brown.
Incubation: in the commonly kept species, both sexes usually incubate for 13 or 14 days.

A pair of bulbuls should live together without fighting, and if they are given their own well-planted aviary, the chances of breeding are good. But in mixed company, some pairs may become aggressive toward others and need to be removed. A cup-shaped nest is constructed, sometimes in an open or half-open-fronted box, but more often in bushes and trees. Grasses, roots, fibers, mosses, dry leaves and animal hair are all used to make a neat or rough nest, depending on the species.

The chicks receive only live food for about the first week, with the adult food included thereafter. Provide the parents with mealworms, waxworms and small crickets for this important period.

The chicks should fledge after about 14 days and become independent 2 or 3 weeks later. Remove the youngsters as soon as they are feeding themselves, because the adults sometimes become aggressive if they wish to renest.

Starlings, Mynahs and Oxpeckers

Order: Passeriformes
Family: Sturnidae

Sturnidae comprises about 108 species that are divided into 2 subfamilies: Sturninae and Buphaginae. One hundred and six species of starlings and mynahs make up Sturninae, while 2 species of tickbirds or oxpeckers comprise Buphaginae.

Starlings

They are distributed throughout the Old World, and the common starling, *Sturnus vulgaris*, can be found almost worldwide. Some starlings are arboreal fruit eaters that live in the jungle and rain forest. But most are insect eaters that spend much of their time on the ground in fairly open country, from forest and forest edge to grassland. Their plumage is often a glossy green, blue or purple, and the head is sometimes crested, with bare skin and/or wattles. Many starlings are gregarious and noisy, and roost in flocks.

The common starling is a fairly typical member of Sturnidae that originated in Europe; but following deliberate introductions it can now be found in South Africa, Australia, New Zealand, Hawaii, North America and elsewhere. Indeed, the millions of common starlings in the United States and Canada are descended from just 60 that were released in New York's Central Park in 1890, and 40 more in 1891. More than a dozen attempts to introduce the common starling had previously failed, but from 1891 the species prospered and was first seen in California in the 1940s.

Nowadays, the common starling is providing a new field of interest, mainly in Europe—color mutations. There are several, such as the "agate" which has light brown wings and a lighter black body than normal; and "isabel" where all of the black on the body is replaced with medium brown while still retaining the white flecks and spangling of the normal. There are near-white varieties and others such as the "opal" and "lace-wing." Many more are likely in the future as work continues to develop new mutations and improve the existing ones.

Mynahs

The names starling, mynah and grackle are very often used interchangeably, and in fact many of the mynahs look very starlinglike. Mynahs are found in New Guinea, Burma, Thailand, south and central China, parts of Indonesia, and especially India. They are mainly dull brown or black with patches of bare yellow skin on the head. Most species can be seen in lightly forested areas and pasture land, or scavenging in towns and market places. The common mynah, *Acridotheres tristis*, has a great liking for locusts, and has been introduced to southern Africa, Australia and many islands in Polynesia, to control them. But unfortunately the bird itself has become a pest by eating fruit, which is the main food source of mynahs.

Oxpeckers

Oxpeckers use their short legs and sharp claws to grip the hide of cattle, zebras, antelopes, rhinos and other large grazing mammals of the African plains. They feed mainly on flies and ticks that infest the skin, but nowadays their numbers are declining as chemicals are used to rid domestic cattle of their parasites.

Size

Starlings: 6.5–12 in. (16–30 cm); some of the African species are made even longer by tails of up to 13 in. (32.5 cm).
Mynahs: 9–12 in. (22.5–30 cm).
Oxpeckers: 7–7.5 in. (17.5–19 cm).

Compatibility

Many of the sturnids live in flocks and often breed colonially. But during the breeding season their temper can be unpredictable. They generally have the potential to become very aggressive, with the smaller, more timid or unpaired birds being particularly vulnerable. Starlings and mynahs can be kept with equally robust birds such as certain laughing thrushes, especially in very large enclosures. But they often disrupt the nesting of other birds, by poking about in nests or taking nesting material, and they may also rob nests of eggs and chicks. It is therefore best to give a pair of sturnids their own aviary.

The Sulawesi king starling, *Basilornis celebensis*, represents a very special hazard: pairs may kill smaller birds in the vicinity of their nest or young. And newly paired king starlings are prone to attacking each other, with either sex easily capable of inflicting fatal injuries.

Diet

Starlings: most species; meat-biased omnivore diet A, with pinkie mice eaten by some starlings.

The following species are more insectivorous and require 75 percent diet G (see page 53) + 25 percent diced fruits, fed in separate dishes: amethyst or violet starling, *Cinnyricinclus leucogaster*; and members of the genera *Lamprotornis* and *Cosmopsarus*.

The rose-colored starling, *Sturnus roseus*, should be given color food to preserve its pink plumage.

Mynahs: meat-biased omnivore diet A (see page 51), with the occasional whole pinkie mouse.

Oxpeckers: standard insectivore diet G, with the occasional sliced or whole pinkie mouse.

Management

Newly imported birds do not need any special foods and after a period of acclimation are easy to maintain. Once acclimated, they are generally hardy and can be kept outside year-round. Although many will live without heat, it is best to provide them with a warm house during freezing weather and a secure shelter at all times. Starlings and mynahs are usually very active birds and need plenty of space to avoid obesity. In the case of the Sulawesi king starling, space is usually a requisite for a pair to live together amicably.

The royal starling, *Cosmopsarus regius*, is slightly less hardy than other sturnids I have kept, and my preference is to winter it in temperatures of at least 60°F (15.6°C).

Breeding

Sexing: the majority are monomorphic. Females may be slightly smaller, have shorter crests or shorter tails. The amethyst or violet starling is one of the few truly dimorphic species. However, many of the African glossy starlings (genus *Lamprotornis*) can be sexed by the difference in the skin color inside their mouths.

Eggs: 2–6 usually pale blue, plain or spotted brown.

Incubation: 11–18 days, often by both parents.

Even if they have been peaceful throughout the year, most sturnids are bold and potentially aggressive during the breeding season. For the general safety of others, they should be given their own large, well-planted aviary.

The majority of species nest in tree holes abandoned by such birds as parrots, woodpeckers or barbets; and the grosbeak starling, *Scissirostrum dubium*, can even use its strong bill to excavate cavities in soft wood, which has earned it the alternative name of woodpecker starling. Indeed, the protractor muscles in the skull are so well developed that they act as a shock absorber, as in the woodpeckers. Sturnids may also nest in holes in masonry or spaces under the eaves of houses.

In captivity, boxes or hollow logs are normally accepted, and rarely birds may build on trays concealed behind foliage. A parakeet-type box with a round entrance hole of about 2.25 (5.6 cm) in diameter or a half-open-fronted box should be located high up in the aviary; some specimens prefer fairly open locations, while others require seclusion. Nests are normally made of grasses, leaves and sometimes a little mud. Many species have a great preference for small, rounded leaves, such as *Ficus benjamina*.

Live food, such as mealworms and waxworms, are fed to the chicks for about the first 5–7 days, with the adult food included thereafter. Pinkie mice may also be eaten, especially by mynahs. The chicks develop quickly and leave the nest at roughly 18–25 days of age, and are fully independent about 2 weeks later. At this point it is best to remove them, since some species become aggressive following a desire to renest; however, the young may be attacked at any time after they have fledged, and should always be watched.

Hybrids

It is interesting to note the starling hybrids that were accidentally bred in the 1960s at the aviaries of Edward Marshall Boehm, near Trenton, New Jersey: royal, *Cosmopsarus regius*, X superb or spreo, *Lamprotornis superbus*; and rose-colored or rosy pastor, *Sturnus roseus*, X pagoda or black-headed, *Sturnus pagodarum* (Everitt, C. 1973).

References

Everitt, C.: (1973) *Birds of the Edward Marshall Boehm Aviaries*. Edward Marshall Boehm, Inc.

Crows, Magpies and Jays

Order: Passeriformes
Family: Corvidae

The crows, jays and magpies number about 113 species and are found nearly worldwide. Those of the genus *Corvus* are mostly black with some white in a few species. The treepies (genus *Dendrocitta*) are more attractive with rufous, gray, black and white plumage. The green magpies or hunting cissas (genus *Cissa*) are a vibrant green. The blue magpies (genus *Urocissa*) are even more beautiful with considerable amounts of blue plumage, and flowing tails that are far longer than their bodies. Roughly 30 of the corvids (in seven genera) are known as blue or American jays, which occur throughout the Americas from Canada to Argentina.

Corvids are found mainly in open woodland, forests and plains; many use their relatively long legs to walk and hop along the ground, as they search for food. The smaller species tend to forage in the treetops, with some eating only specialized foods such as seeds and nuts. But most are true omnivores, eating fruits, young birds, carrion and almost anything that is edible.

Size

Medium to large birds 8–28 in. (20–70 cm), including the ravens which are the largest passerines. But all of the commonly kept magpies and jays only measure about 14 in. (35 cm), nearly half of which represents the tail.

Compatibility

On the whole, corvids are predatory and not to be trusted with smaller or weaker birds. They can be kept in pairs, and in the wild, some species live and breed in groups, including: the magpie-jays (genus *Calocitta*) and the azure-winged magpie, *Cyanopica cyana*. The 4 *Cissilopha* jays are remarkably sociable year-round, with individuals helping to raise the young of others in the group.

Diet

Diet A (see page 51) for meat-biased omnivores.

Management

These are very hardy birds, and can be kept outside year-round without heat. But they must have access to a frost-free house and are best shut in during severe weather. Newly imported hunting cissas and treepies may need more insects to assist the acclimation process because they are largely insectivorous; but after a short time they should graduate onto diet A without any problems.

In captivity (and indeed in the wild), the green plumage of the hunting cissas can change to blue. Yellow feathers also become white and red feathers become brown. The green appearance is created by the combination of blue and yellow pigment in the feathers. In regions where there is little cover, sunlight "burns out" the yellow, to leave only the blue. This can happen in just a few days, and is remedied by reducing the intensity of artificial lighting or providing more cover. The vibrancy of the plumage will also be affected if there are insufficient yellow carotenoids in the diet.

Certain species from all genera cache foods in times of plenty. In the warmer months this may be a health hazard, and stored food should probably be removed. However, corvids are known for eating their young. Allowing a fresh store of food to remain in the aviary may help satisfy their natural foraging instincts, and perhaps assuage their worst tendencies.

Breeding

Sexing: virtually all are monomorphic.
Eggs: 2–7, usually blue, green or gray with dark markings
Incubation: 16–21 days, normally only by the female, except in the nutcrackers.

Many corvids do not breed until they are 2 years old. And most of the species kept in captivity are solitary nesters, except certain sociable ones mentioned under Compatibility. Thickish sticks usually form the foundation of the nest, on which a cup or bowl of finer grasses and rootlets is built. This is often a bulky structure located in the branches of a tree, and sometimes in a hole in rock work. In captivity, a flat platform or a half-open-fronted box can be offered, preferably high up and in thick vegetation.

Both sexes build the nest and feed the young, and the male feeds the female while she is on the nest. But unlike other passerines, food is not carried in the bill; instead it is held in the throat or a small pouch within the chin, called the sublingual pouch.

Sometimes corvids eat their young, which can be a difficult problem to cure once it has become habitual. Perhaps in the aviary, because they are denied the natural activity of foraging and making caches, these intelligent birds become bored and turn on their young. Try to increase their foraging activity by placing small amounts of food around the aviary; burying foods in a tray of bran makes the search seem more realistic.

The parents will need additional insects and meats, such as pinkie mice, to feed the growing family. And once the young of most species are independent, it is best to remove them from the aviary, in case their parents attack them.

Oropendolas

Order: Passeriformes
Family: Icteridae
Subfamily: Icterinae

There are 12 oropendola species that represent a small part of the family of New World blackbirds. They are the largest of the icterids and share the same general build and appearance of the caciques, to which they are closely related. The oropendolas are not colorful, being predominantly green, black or chestnut. But they are exceptionally impressive looking: all have bright yellow tails and fearsome, pointed conical bills that are topped at the forehead with a prominent swelling. Most species are fairly common and live in flocks of at least 20, with far greater numbers congregating to roost.

Oropendolas can be found in every country in Central and South America except Uruguay, Chile and parts of the Guianas; and the crested oropendola, *Psarocolius decumanus insularis*, can even be found on the islands of Trinidad and Tobago. Oropendolas usually inhabit fairly open areas such as marshes, clearings and the forest edge, and in summer certain species ascend up to 6,500 ft. (1,950 m). They are permanent residents of the tropics; and colonies of oropendolas make themselves conspicuous by building long, pendantlike nests in isolated trees. They spend much of their time in the canopy of humid, dense forest, eating fruits, insects, nectar and almost any small animal prey they can find.

Size

Largest: montezuma, *Psarocolius montezuma*, male 20 in. (50 cm and 520 g), female 15 in. (38 cm and 230 g).

Smallest: band-tailed, *P. latirostris*, male 12 in. (30 cm and 190 g), female 8 in. (20 cm and 105 g).

Compatibility

These are sociable birds, and colonies normally have more females than males. Two oropendola species sometimes share the same nesting or roosting tree, but generally one species will take a tree for itself and not mix with others.

In the aviary, oropendolas should not be kept with smaller birds, since their large bills and mostly omnivorous feeding habits could result in injuries or robbed nests. One male and 2 or 3 females should be given their own, very large aviary.

Diet

Meat-biased omnivore diet A (see page 51), and an occasional pinkie mouse.

The yellow tail feathers can fade after successive molts in captivity, and yellow carotenoids are recommended in the diet.

Management

Provided they are healthy, oropendolas are the easiest of birds to acclimate from the wild. They are tough and willing to sample new foods, and individuals tend to settle down very quickly.

Acclimated birds are hardy and can live outside year-round. During freezing weather they should be shut into a frost-free house; and although it is not absolutely essential, some warmth for the coldest periods is beneficial.

Breeding

Sexing: dimorphic, males have brighter plumage, are roughly twice the weight of females and are up to 50 percent longer.

Eggs: usually 2 perhaps 3, pale with dark spots, lines and blotches.

Incubation: solely by the female; 17 or 18 days for the crested oropendola, *Psarocolius decumanus*, fledging at 31–36 days.

Oropendolas breed in colonies, building up to 100 nests in tall, clearly visible trees. Their nests are caciquelike, being long sleeves of plant fibers, mosses or palm leaves that hang from the end of a branch. They are normally 3–6 ft. long (0.9–1.8 m) with the entrance at the top; the nest chamber is at the bottom and is often lined with small leaves.

Breeding is polygynous, where females outnumber males. Females nest-build, incubate and rear the young completely by themselves, while the males stand guard at the top of the tree. After leaving the nest, young oropendolas fly about in flocks and can be fed by the accompanying females for weeks before they are fully independent.

Bee Eaters

Order: Coraciiformes
Family: Meropidae

These are large-headed, long-billed and very beautiful birds. In most of the approximately 23 species, the plumage is green with shades of red, yellow, black, blue or rufous. Tails are normally long with elongated central feathers, and facial patterns are distinctive, often sporting a black mask that makes the bill seem greater and more formidable.

Bee eaters are insectivorous, eating mainly flying insects, although the carmine bee eater, *Merops nubicus*, does have a distinct penchant for grasshoppers and locusts. In its search for food, the carmine will actually ride on the backs of animals, such as ostriches, antelopes, elephants and warthogs, waiting to catch any insects that are flushed out. Equally unusual is the white-throated bee eater, *Merops albicollis*, the only member of Meropidae to eat vegetable matter. In the rain forests of West Africa, squirrels feed on oil-palm nuts by first peeling off the skin. As the oily skins flutter down, the waiting bee eaters catch, and eat them.

Most bee eaters avoid heavy forest, preferring lightly wooded or open country; and they are normally found where food is abundant, near rivers, swamps, lakes, coastal mangroves and flooded rice fields. Bee eaters typically perch on fences, telegraph wires and branches, waiting to chase virtually any airborne insect, which can be as far away as 300 ft. (91 m). All species can eat dangerous insects such as bees, wasps and hornets, which are rendered harmless before being eaten: the tail (and sting) of the insect is vigorously rubbed against the perch; this causes the expression of the venom and often the sting itself.

Local, seasonal movements of bee eaters are fairly common, and a few species migrate many thousands of miles. The European bee eater, *Merops apiaster*, and blue-cheeked bee eater, *M. superciliosus*, breed in Europe and Asia, and migrate to Africa for the winter; the Australian bee eater, *M. ornatus*, winters in the Lesser Sunda Islands and breeds in Australia. Most species can be found in North Africa, with a handful in the Middle East, Asia and Southeast Asia.

Size

These are total measurements that include long tails and often even longer streamers.

White-throated: 11 in. (28 cm); the body is very small and only weighs about 20 grams.

Carmine: One of the largest species at 14 in. (35 cm). The smallest species is the little bee eater, *Merops pusillus*, at only 6 in. (15 cm).

Compatibility

Red-bearded, *Nyctyornis amicta*, and blue-bearded bee eaters, *N. athertoni*, live singly or in pairs. Carmine bee eaters live in small groups, and gather in their hundreds or thousands to breed. Generally, bee eaters are fairly sociable birds that can be kept in small groups and with similar-sized, nonaggressive species. However, they are far less likely to tolerate others during the breeding season; and breeding pairs can become so aggressive toward all other birds they have to be given their own aviary.

Diet

Diet H (see page 54) for difficult insectivores. Color food is essential for most species, to preserve the red, yellow and orange plumage. It is normal for bee eaters to cast up pellets of undigested food, like a bird of prey; the process is facilitated by the bird bashing its bill against the perch.

Management

Like all insectivores, it is fairly easy to sustain bee eaters for a few weeks on mealworms and waxworms. But long-term success can only be achieved by successfully transferring the birds onto a more nutritious (artificial) diet as urgently as possible. This can be a laborious process, and should only be undertaken by the most experienced aviculturists.

Acclimated and established bee eaters are not hard to keep and in warm climates do very well outdoors, adoring the occasional warm shower and the opportunity to sunbathe. In temperate climates, a heated house is essential, since bee eaters must be protected from cold weather and persistent rain. They will often stand out in the rain to the point of being saturated, sick and unable to fly.

Bee eaters have relatively long wings, and should be provided with large, fairly open aviaries. Food dishes must be raised several feet above the ground, and positioned in the open so the birds can feed while hovering. Bee eaters will live with other birds, although my preference is to give them their own aviary; this minimizes food competition, helping the shier birds to get the range of foods vital for good health.

Breeding

Sexing: virtually all species are monomorphic. The red-bearded, *Nyctyornis amicta*, is dimorphic.

Eggs: white; 2–5 in the tropics. Clutch size increases at higher latitudes, and bee eaters in Eurasia can lay as many as 10 eggs.

Incubation: usually shared by both sexes for 18–22 days.

Bee eaters lay their eggs in an unlined chamber at the end of a tunnel. It is dug in a sandy or earth bank, or even in the ground, and for carmine bee eaters measures 3–7 ft. long (0.9–2.1 m) and about 2.5 in. (6 cm) wide. Holes may be dug some time before nesting begins, and several attempts at digging may be made until a satisfactory burrow is completed. Nests can be used for several years, becoming very smelly, or the birds may go elsewhere and start afresh.

In captivity, the best breeding results are achieved if the birds are allowed to dig their own burrow, very preferably into a perpendicular surface. To help stimulate breeding activity, maggots can be allowed to metamorphose into flies within the aviary, and generally the live food content of the diet can be increased by about 20 percent.

When I was a boy, I kept 7 carmine bee eaters of unknown sex in an aviary 15 ft. (4.5 m) square. Against one side of the aviary I built a large wooden box 6 ft. (1.8 m) square and 4 ft. (1.2 m) deep, which was heavily reinforced on all sides. The sides and back were covered with plywood; the front was partly open and covered with ten-gauge wire mesh. The box was filled with equal parts of soil, sand and peat moss, and had sheets of thin plywood running horizontally through it to help protect the tunnels from collapse. At the front of the box, parts of the wire mesh were cut away to expose the soil mixture; and to encourage tunneling, holes 2 in. (5 cm) deep were started in the soil.

In the first year, the birds dug only one hole to a depth of about 10 in. (25 cm). In the second year, two new holes were dug to a depth of about 3 ft. (0.9 m); there was a tiny chamber at the end of one, but no eggs were laid. In May of the following year, another 3 ft. tunnel was dug, which had a larger chamber—each tunnel was almost perfectly straight and level. Incubation started soon after the tunnel was complete, but no chicks emerged. Later inspection revealed 3 clear eggs.

Rollers

Order: Coraciiformes
Family: Coraciidae

Rollers are named for their stunning, rolling and tumbling displays, seen mostly during courtship and often accompanied by grating screams. There are twelve species in Coraciidae, comprising 2 genera: *Coracias* and *Eurystomus*. The 8 *Coracias* rollers include the more familiar avicultural species such as the European, *C. garrulus*; lilac-breasted, *C. caudata*; Indian blue, *C. benghalensis*; and racquet-tailed, *C. spatulata*.

Rollers tend to live singly or in pairs, congregating in groups where food is abundant. Both of the African *Eurystomus* species may even gather in the tens of thousands to exploit swarms of flying ants and termites. Rollers are capable of taking food on the wing or from the ground. But in general, *Eurystomus* species prefer to catch, and eat, insects on the wing, while *Coracias* rollers tend to prey on small ground animals. Almost anything is eaten, including scorpions, small snakes, lizards, rodents, worms, mollusks and young birds, and very rarely, fish.

Rollers inhabit fairly open country and can often be seen on exposed perches by the roadside, or in areas of cultivation. They come from southern Europe, the Middle East, Australia and throughout Asia and North Africa.

Size

Fairly stocky birds: 10–15 in. (25–38 cm).

Compatibility

Rollers can usually be kept in pairs. They will live with similarly sized, arboreal birds, although slow fledglings are vulnerable and easily eaten.

Diet

New birds may have to be carefully acclimated using diet H (see page 54) and the meating-off techniques described earlier. Established birds can then graduate onto diet G (page 53), which should include large crickets and mealworms, with a small mouse, lizard, frog or pieces of lean meat, added each day. If the birds will eat them, small balls of Nebraska Bird of Prey Diet are also excellent.

Management

In captivity, rollers can become quite sluggish, but in the company of other, largish birds they are more active and alert. Most species enjoy bathing and especially sunbathing, and do best in large aviaries where they can exercise properly. Established birds are fairly hardy, although they must be protected from heavy rain and cold weather; heated winter accommodation is therefore important.

Breeding

Sexing: monomorphic.
Eggs: 2–6 white.
Incubation: usually by both sexes, Indian blue 17–19 days; lilac-breasted 22–24 days; European 18–19 days.

Rollers almost always nest in holes, either in a tree or in the masonry of a wall or house. Old woodpecker and barbet nests may also be used. Occasionally, lilac-breasted rollers build their nests in termite mounds. Most species line the nest with feathers, grasses, dead leaves or pieces of old rag.

In captivity, rollers should be given the largest possible aviary, so they can more easily complete their courtship flights. Nest boxes will usually be accepted, and designs with a round entrance hole or a half-open front should be offered. Position both types of boxes as high as possible and in secluded corners.

Chicks are usually reared by both parents and fledge at about 1 month of age. Provide plenty of live food such as waxworms, mealworms, pinkie mice and large crickets; all should be dusted with a multivitamin and mineral supplement.

Hornbills

Order: Coraciiformes
Family: Bucerotidae

With their long, decurved bills and omnivorous feeding habits, hornbills are the toucans of the Old World. There are about 48 species, many of which have a prominent casque on top of their bill. This is normally a lightweight, honeycombed (partly hollow) structure, that may help to reinforce the bill or act as a shock absorber while nest cavities are being modified.

Hornbills live in the tropical evergreen forests of Asia and Southeast Asia, and in the forests and savanna of sub-Saharan Africa.

They are mostly arboreal and eat large amounts of fruit, especially figs, and may gather in feeding parties of over 100 at fruiting trees. But members of the genus *Tockus* spend a lot of time foraging on the ground and are fairly insectivorous, while the two ground hornbills (genus *Bucorvus*) are completely terrestrial and virtually carnivorous, preying upon insects, rats, mice, small birds, eggs and snakes. Hornbills do not drink very much, if at all, and normally obtain sufficient water from their food.

Several hornbill species live in groups, with the members jointly defending a territory and often helping the dominant (alpha) pair to feed their young. However, the majority of hornbills seem to live in pairs, where the birds usually forage independently of each other.

Size

The great Indian hornbill, *Buceros bicornis*, is the largest at 52 in. (130 cm).

Small species such as the red-billed, *Tockus erythrorhynchus*, and yellow billed, *T. flavirostris,* measure about 18 in. (45 cm).

Compatibility

Given their feeding habits, hornbills are obviously a potential hazard in a mixed collection, with the larger species capable of eating small birds, and all species capable of eating fledglings. Hornbills can be kept with similar-sized birds, but generally it is far better to give a pair their own aviary.

Diet

Ground hornbills: diet I (see page 56) for carnivores. Other species: diet A (page 51) for meat-biased omnivores. A chopped or whole mouse can also be added to the diet every 2 or 3 days, and more often to help achieve breeding condition. Hornbills swallow their food whole, so it is important to provide foods they can pick up and swallow easily—chop fruits and meats into bite-sized pieces.

Management

Hornbills are robust and impressive birds that are fairly easy to keep. The smaller species do not require particularly large aviaries although the bigger hornbills should certainly be given as much space as possible.

In temperate climates, large hornbills can live outdoors year-round, and do not need any heat if they are given a good quality, frost-free house. But the smaller species tend to be less hardy and should be shut into a heated house during wintery weather.

Breeding

Sexing: great Indian, dimorphic. Male, red eyes; female, white eyes. Yellow-billed, monomorphic. Red-billed, monomorphic. However, the male may have more black on lower mandible.

Eggs: small species lay up to 6 eggs; large species lay 2 eggs. All species lay white eggs.

Incubation: small species approximately 25 days; large species approximately 45 days.

Pairs do not always live together amicably, but if all is well, increased vocalizations, displaying, courtship-feeding and beak clacking should be the prelude to breeding. Hornbills nest in cavities in trees or rock work. In captivity, nest boxes (up to 2 m tall for large species) are usually accepted and can be enhanced by fixing bark pieces to the exterior; or an old tree trunk can be used, once it has been excavated to make a large cavity.

The nesting female must be able to easily look out of the nest cavity; this helps her to see and dispatch predators, and it also allows the male to pass food to her. To meet this requirement the cavity should contain a sufficient depth of wood shavings, to which the adults may add leaves, flowers, grasses or even small rocks. If the log is soft or rotten enough, the birds will probably add their own substrate by hammering the cavity roof and walls.

The shape and size of the cavity entrance hole is also very important. The hole should only be slightly wider than the birds' shoulder width, and of an upright, oval shape. This is because the female of all species, except the ground hornbills, is sealed into the cavity by a wall of feces, sticky fruits, nest debris and mud. If the hole in the nest log is too wide, the birds will be unable to plaster it in and breeding will not take place. But if all goes well, the female is plastered into the cavity and fed by the male through a narrow slit.

In the wild, ground hornbills also use tree cavities. However, in captivity such birds cannot usually fly (having been pinioned or wing-clipped) and need assistance to breed. Captive birds have been known to nest on the ground behind a large log. But normally a box or tree cavity is provided, and stood on the ground or fixed slightly above it. Ground hornbills do not mud-in the entrance hole as with all other hornbills; the shape and size of the hole is therefore not as important and can be fairly large.

In most species of large forest hornbills, the females stay in the nest until the chicks are ready to fledge. But with other hornbills (such as *Tockus* species) the female emerges far earlier to help gather food for the growing family. At this point the young reseal the hole themselves, using feces and food remains.

Incubation starts with the laying of the first egg; and with small species (that have as many as 6 eggs) this can mean an age difference of well over a week between the oldest and youngest chick.

The older chicks therefore have the best chances of survival, unless there are birds from the previous year's breeding that can help rear the new family. Even species that only have 2 eggs may fail to rear both chicks, and in captivity it can be very beneficial to consider hand rearing the youngest bird or birds.

When chicks are in the nest, special foods are not necessary. But be sure to provide plenty of soft foods such as juicy fruits, large insects, and chopped and whole pinkie mice. All should be dusted with a multivitamin and mineral supplement, and chopped smaller than usual so that the chicks can safely swallow them.

Kingfishers and Kookaburras

Order: Coraciiformes
Family: Alcedinidae

Kingfishers can be divided into 2 broad groups: the fishing kingfishers that feed on fish, crustaceans and aquatic insects, and depend on water for their living; and the forest kingfishers that have lost their reliance on water, and eat insects, rodents, small birds and lizards. The fishing kingfishers (subfamilies Cerylinae and Alcedininae) have sharp, daggerlike bills, whereas the forest species (subfamily Daceloninae) have broader, hook-tipped bills, that are better suited for grasping and crushing prey.

The laughing kookaburra, *Dacelo novaeguineae*, and bluewinged kookaburra, *D. leachii*, are among the most well known of the forest kingfishers, being highly predatory and capable of eating snakes of up to 3 ft. (0.9 m) long. Many of the *Halcyon* species are also forest kingfishers, that rarely if ever feed at water, but instead live on insects and ground animals. Some kingfishers are intermediate between the aquatic and forest lifestyles, like most of the *Ceyx* species, which are capable of catching insects on the wing, but will also eat tadpoles and frogs from small pools.

Kingfishers tend to avoid open country, and keep to waterways or tropical rain forest, depending on their feeding habits. They nearly always hunt from one particular perch, flying or diving at their prey. And some fishing species (of the subfamily Cerylinae) have also developed the ability to hover, kestrel-like, over water, enabling them to hunt far offshore. The approximately 92 kingfisher species are almost cosmopolitan; the majority live in Southeast Asia and Indonesia, with only 6 species being found in the New World.

Size

Small to medium: 4–18 in. (10–45 cm).

Compatibility

Kingfishers normally live singly or in pairs; and some species, such as the laughing kookaburra, can live in family units, with each member helping to incubate, and rear the young. In captivity, a newly formed pair of mature kingfishers may be aggressive toward each other, whereas pairing them before the age of 8 months old is usually successful. Kingfishers can be kept with other robust birds of similar size.

Diet

Forest kingfishers, and species intermediate between insectivore and piscivore (genera *Ceyx*, *Tanysiptera*, *Halcyon*): 60 percent diet G + 40 percent diet I, including large crickets, large mealworms, small fish and small mice ("pinkie" or "fuzzy"). Mix all ingredients together.

True fishing species (subfamilies Cerylinae and Alcedininae): 30 percent diet G (see page 53) + 70 percent diet I, including small fish, frogs and lizards. Acclimating such birds from the wild is exceedingly hard, which is why they are very rarely seen in captivity—a pool with live fish is almost essential.

Kookaburras: diet I for carnivores. It is normal for kingfishers to cast up a pellet of undigested food, like bee eaters and birds of prey.

Management

Kingfishers are not very good at maneuvering, or even stopping, in a small space; and generally they do best in large, tall and fairly secluded aviaries.

Kookaburras can live outside year-round without heat. But they must always have access to a shelter and be shut into a frost-free house during severe weather. All of the other kingfisher species should be provided with heat during cold weather, along with a night light to enable all night feeding.

Breeding

Sexing: blue-winged kookaburra; dimorphic. The tail is blue in male, red-brown in female.

Laughing kookaburra; should be considered monomorphic. Differences between sexes are not definitive.

White-collared kingfisher; should be considered monomorphic. Differences in coloration are only obvious when two birds can be compared.

Gray-headed kingfisher; monomorphic.

Eggs: usually 2 or 3 in the tropics, and up to 10 at higher latitudes; all species lay white eggs.

Incubation: 17–27 days.

The fishing kingfishers of Cerylinae and Alcedininae nest in tunnels that they usually excavate themselves in earthen banks, often at the edge of water. Some of the forest species also nest in earthen burrows, although they normally use tree holes. If the wood is sufficiently soft, they will excavate the cavity themselves, otherwise an old barbet, parakeet or woodpecker hole is equally acceptable. Several species also burrow into arboreal termite mounds.

Nest boxes are usually accepted, either with a half-open front or a round entrance hole (slightly wider than the birds' shoulder width). They should be filled with several centimeters of wood shavings and positioned as high as possible in the aviary. Kingfishers do not take nesting material to the box, but lay their eggs directly onto the shavings. The same box is often used year-after-year.

Initially, the chicks are fed mealworms, waxworms and crickets. But very quickly the parents start to feed pinkie mice and small fish; and once the young are only 2 to 4 days old, both adults spend increasingly longer periods away from the nest. The rearing foods should be sprinkled with a multivitamin and mineral supplement to ensure healthy growth.

Toucans, Toucanets and Aracaris

Order: Piciformes
Family: Ramphastidae

With their huge, colorful and often serrated bills, toucans are unmistakable and wonderful. There are about 35 species, all of which are arboreal inhabitants of the rain forests and wooded areas of tropical America. They are largely frugivorous and use their long bills to reach forward and pluck berries from thin, fragile twigs, showing a preference for dry, fibrous fruits such as *Ficus* berries. But meat is also included in the diet, and toucans will prey upon nestlings, lizards, small rodents and even small snakes. For its size, the bill is very lightweight, and can be used quite deftly; in cross section it looks like a mass of cobwebs, loosely molded together and covered with a protective skin.

Toucans, toucanets and aracaris often live in loose flocks of five to ten, and usually keep to the upper levels of the forest. Most do not come to the ground, and drink from rain-filled hollows high up in the branches. Ramphastids live in Mexico and Central America; and they range throughout the entire northern part of South America, mostly at lower altitudes, although a few species can be found in the Andes.

Size

Toco toucan, *Ramphastos toco*, is the largest species at 24 in. (60 cm), including the bill which measures up to 7.5 in. (19 cm) long. Toucanets and aracaris are smaller at 10–15 in. (25–38 cm).

Compatibility

Pairs of the smaller toucans (aracaris or toucanets) can be kept with robust, similar-sized birds like magpies and large laughing thrushes. I have kept a pair of channel-billed toucans, *Ramphastos vitellinus*, with Pekin robins, silver-eared mesias and stilts. But when the breeding season approaches, ramphastids are likely to become aggressive, with most of them capable of inflicting harm; and at any time they may eat the nestlings of other birds. It is therefore best to give a pair their own aviary, especially for the largest and most dangerous of all, the toco toucan. The only exceptions are the toucanets, which are safe with similar-sized birds, even when breeding.

Newly introduced pairs of ramphastids can sometimes be very aggressive toward each other. If possible both birds should be released into a new aviary together, so that neither has a territorial advantage. If you are introducing a new bird to an established one, catch the old bird from its aviary and put it in a box. Add new perches to the enclosure to make it look like a new aviary and release both birds together. The established bird should be as confused as the newcomer and hopefully they will settle down together—the chances of success are far greater if you can introduce an immature pair.

Diet

Diet B (see page 51) for fruit-biased omnivores. A small amount of raw meat, such as a chopped or whole mouse, lean hamburger or balls of Bird of Prey Diet, can also be fed every 2 or 3 days. Live food such as mealworms and crickets may be eaten, especially by the smaller species.

The food should be chopped into cubes or rolled into balls so that it is easy to pick up and swallow. Toucans are not capable of tearing up their food and either swallow it whole, or do not eat it at all.

Virtually all ramphastids are well known for being susceptible to iron-storage disease, and low iron softbill pellets are recommended.

Management

Thoroughly acclimated and established, these birds are hardy and can be kept outdoors. But even established birds can suffer from the cold, and rarely the beak can be damaged by frost. Toucans should therefore be shut into a heated shelter during wintery nights and severe weather.

Toucans are very active birds and require a large, fairly high aviary with a few stout perches placed as far from each other as possible. This encourages exercise by flying, instead of simply bouncing from branch to branch. Plants are very useful in any breeding aviary, but toucans tend to be quite destructive to most plantlife; and the toughest varieties, such as conifers, are recommended—a carpet of grass, however, usually thrives unmolested.

Perching should have fairly sharp, rigid spikes which toucans use to clean the inside of the upper mandible. Food deposits can otherwise accumulate and turn bad (Seibels, B. 1996).

Breeding

Sexing: all species are monomorphic, except certain aracaris and toucanets of the genus *Selenidera* (females mostly chestnut on underparts). Generally, males are larger bodied with longer bills, but this may be variable and cannot be considered definitive.

Eggs: 2–4 white.

Incubation: all species 16 days (Jennings, J. 1996).

All of the toucans nest in tree holes, such as old woodpecker cavities for the smaller species, and macaw nests for the larger ones. Holes in rotten trees may also be occupied; but toucans are not able to excavate their nests as such, and can only modify the walls or entrance hole where the wood is soft.

Tall nest boxes or hollowed-out palm logs should be fixed as high as possible in the aviary. The nest cavity should be about 10 in. (25 cm) diameter for toco toucans and at least 7 in. (18 cm) for other toucan species. And aracaris (genus *Pteroglossus*) often use their boxes for roosting, where groups will huddle together for the night.

Toucans lay their eggs in an unlined cavity; both sexes usually incubate and rear the young. The chicks develop very slowly: fledging occurs at about 4 to 6 weeks in the smaller species, and 7 weeks or more in the toco toucan. Young ramphastids have amazing, ridged heel pads which help them move about in the nest cavity.

Plenty of soft fruits are required as a rearing food; these should be chopped into small cubes that the young can safely swallow. To provide sufficient protein for the growing chicks, foods such as mealworms, large crickets, balls of meat, pinkie mice, frogs and lizards can also be given.

Toucans can be hand reared using the techniques described in the Hand Rearing section. But they are susceptible to *Candida* infections. If treated with Nystatin, these can be prevented fairly easily, otherwise death is invariably the result. (See Ailments—Candidiasis.)

References

Jennings, J. *AFA Watchbird*, vol. XXIII, no.2, March/April 1996. The Collared Aracari.

Seibels, B. Personal communication. 1996.

Barbets

Order: Piciformes
Family: Capitonidae

The barbets are a tropical family of about 80 species, with a distribution affecting South America, Asia and Africa. They are mostly arboreal, forest and woodland birds, although some of the African species live in arid scrublands. Barbets have stocky bodies, large heads and powerful beaks, which have beardlike bristles at their base. It is these bristles that provide the common name since "barbet" means bearded. Their legs are short and feet are zygodactyl: two toes pointing forward and two back; and because their wings are short and rounded, flight is relatively weak. A few barbet species have quite pleasant whistling calls, although the vast majority utter shrill and monotonous sounds, often for very long periods.

Size

The tinkerbirds (genus *Pogoniulus*) from Africa represent the smallest barbets at only about 3.5 in. (9 cm), while the giant barbet, *Megalaima virens*, from Southeast Asia measures 13 in. (33 cm) long.

Compatibility

Barbets can be aggressive to birds of equal or lesser size, and most, if not all, species will rob nests of young chicks. Male barbets may be very aggressive toward their mate, and a temporary separation is sometimes necessary. A large, densely planted aviary can help such pairs live together more successfully; and generally, the larger the aviary, the better.

Diet

Asian and African species: meat-biased omnivore diet A (see page 51).

South American species: fruit-biased omnivore diet B (see page 51).

The reds and yellows of many barbets tend to fade in captivity, and a color food is recommended. (See Color Foods.)

Management

In spite of their robust appearance, newly imported barbets may be difficult to establish, and smaller species should be considered delicate, especially the coppersmith, *Megalaima haemacephala*; pied, *Tricholaema leucomelaina*; and flame-headed, *Eubucco bourcierii*. Many barbets need a nest box, which they sleep in and often use as a retreat. Barbets can be kept in outdoor aviaries, but heated winter accommodation must be provided since they are only half hardy; and all species are especially susceptible to damp and drafts.

Breeding

Sexing: in most species the sexes are similar or the same.

Eggs: 2–4 white eggs are laid directly on the wood chips and debris of the nesting chamber.

Incubation: 12–19 days.

In the wild, barbets usually excavate a nest hole in the trunk or bough of a dead or soft-wood tree. But a minority of African species, such as the red and yellow barbet, *Trachyphonus erythrocephalus*, excavate holes in the ground or in termite mounds. If suitable trees are not available, the pied barbet, *Tricholaema leucomelaina*, will even use the grass nests of the sociable weaver, *Philetairus socius*.

In captivity, chances of success are best when the birds are able to excavate their own nest cavity, in a semirotten or soft-wood log. The tunnel to the cavity can be 12 in. (30 cm) long, and so logs should be as wide as possible and up to 7 ft. (2.1 m) tall. Palm logs are ideal and can be stood upright or at an angle. They should be positioned at various heights in the aviary, as well as on the floor; and to encourage breeding, 1 or 2 holes can be started in the side of the logs, facing away from any possible disturbance. Nest boxes are also worth trying, and will need to be a similar size to the logs. Rough pieces of wood and bark should be fixed to the interior and exterior of the box. This will help stimulate natural hammering and excavating activities, and hopefully promote breeding.

Plenty of mealworms, waxworms and crickets will be needed as a rearing food. As the chicks grow, small pinkie mice and soft fruits (including soaked sultanas) form an increasing part of their diet.

Hummingbirds

Order: Apodiformes
Family: Trochilidae

This New World family of well over 300 species is confined mainly to the tropics of Central and South America, with several species ranging into the United States and Canada. The rufous hummingbird, *Selasphorus rufus*, can even be found in southeastern Alaska, from where it migrates more than 3,500 miles to Mexico, for the winter. This is just one of many astounding features of Trochilidae.

The smaller species have a wing beat of nearly 80 per second in forward flight and can travel up to 40 mph (65 kph); and nearly 200 wing beats per second in courtship dives, reaching 59 mph (95 kph).

The breast muscle accounts for up to 30 percent of total body weight, allowing the wings to be as powerful moving up, as they are moving down. The entire wing is able to rotate at the shoulder joint, enabling total flight-control, prolonged hovering and backward flight.

The normal body temperature of an active hummingbird is 104°F (40°C). But when food is short, some hummingbirds are capable of going into a nightly state of torpor. This is where the body temperature falls to as low as 64°F (18°C), with an equally reduced heart and respiration rate. In this way, energy consumption is greatly reduced and certain species are able to eke out a living in cold environments, and almost up to the snow line in the Andes.

Size

The smallest bird in the world is the bee hummingbird, *Calypte helenae*; 2.4 in. (6 cm), weighing 1/15 oz (2 g). The largest hummingbird is the giant, *Patagona gigas*; 8 in. (20 cm).

Compatibility

There is considerable variation between different species and specimens. A great many are quite safe with other hummingbirds, although males can sometimes be aggressive; and when the breeding season approaches, problems can almost be guaranteed. The key to keeping, and breeding, groups of hummingbirds in 1 enclosure is space. Twenty or more birds (of both sexes and 2 or 3 species) may be kept together, provided the enclosure is planted and at least 30 ft. (9 m) square; this should give enough space for each bird to establish its own territory.

Diet

Diet D (see page 52) for hummingbirds. Prepare fresh nectar each day and feed the hummingbirds twice a day. Be sure to thoroughly clean the feeding tubes and let them completely dry out before they are used again: dirty feeding utensils are a primary cause of illness in nectivores, and it is far easier to prevent disease than cure it, especially in such minute birds.

Management

Thanks to the proprietary nectars that are readily available, the hardest part of keeping hummingbirds has been done for us. But their food and feeding habits still need very careful attention, and if neglected the birds can quickly deteriorate.

Nowadays, newly imported birds are not often seen. But if they become available, each bird must be quarantined individually and, preferably, visually separated from the others. A plant sprayer can also be used to spray tepid water on the birds to help improve their plumage. Generally, all hummingbirds must be allowed to bathe regularly to maintain their flying ability and therefore their health. Leaves of plants should be sprayed so that the birds may bathe on them, shallow water dishes should always be available, and a plant sprayer can be used to rain water droplets onto a perching bird—only do this if it is welcomed by the hummingbird.

Newly imported hummingbirds are often infected with *Candida* and must be treated with Nystatin. The easiest method is to treat the nectar. However, in severe cases the mouth can be so full of the fungus that the bill cannot properly close; and the Nystatin has to be painted directly onto the fungus with a small artist's brush. Up to about 10 percent of a hummingbird shipment may be severely infected and curing such birds is difficult. Even specimens that look well can be infected, and so in the case of newly imported hummingbirds, using Nystatin on a prophylactic basis can be very helpful. I would certainly recommend treating the entire shipment the moment *Candida* is detected. (See Ailments—Candidiasis.)

When adding a new hummingbird to your collection, be sure to use the same brand of nectar as that used by the bird's previous owner. Or change from the old to the new food gradually to prevent causing a digestive disturbance and enteritis. (See Sunbirds and Spiderhunters—management.)

Acclimated hummingbirds are surprisingly hardy and easily tolerate temperatures as low as 60°F (16°C); in general the South American species are best kept at 65°–70°F (18°–21°C). The sparkling violet-ear, *Colibri coruscans* (and the 3 other *Colibri* species) are particularly hardy and suitable for the newcomer to hummingbird aviculture, although they can be unusually pugnacious toward other hummingbirds. Likewise, the 31 species of the genus *Amazilia* are fairly hardy, easy to establish and do well in captivity; but many are also quite aggressive, and neither genera should be kept in groups.

Breeding

Sexing: in most species males are more colorful, often with decorations such as gorgets (iridescent throat patches), crowns and long tails.

Eggs: 2, white
Incubation: 14–21 days

In captivity, a pair of hummingbirds should live together year-round if they are given a large enough enclosure. But if there are any problems with aggression, they can be housed in adjacent aviaries within sight of each other; and very preferably they should be separated by a completely removable partition. Hopefully, the female will start to show an interest in the nesting materials and begin nest-building. At this point remove the partition so that both birds can move freely around the entire enclosure.

The female builds the nest alone and some time before copulation. The design and location of the nest varies greatly according to the species, and can be secured to a horizontal branch, a rock wall or suspended by thin strands. In captivity, various materials can be used, such as strips of tissue paper, cotton, animal hair, feathers and cotton wool. Bark, moss and lichens may also be used to camouflage the exterior of the nest, as well as cobwebs to wrap around the structure and secure it to a solid substrate.

Incubation normally begins with the laying of the first egg. The female feeds the chicks on a regurgitated mixture of nectar and a considerable number of tiny insects, such as fruit flies. In the wild, males of most (if not all) species leave the female soon after copulation. In captivity, his continued presence during incubation can be a distraction and a nuisance, and he may have to be removed. Once the chicks are independent, the female sometimes chases them away in an effort to defend her food source; and for their own safety they may have to be separated.

Rails

Order: Gruiformes
Family: Rallidae

There are approximately 124 species in this family, which includes the crakes, coots and gallinules (or moorhens). They are ground-dwelling birds, although some roost in trees and are good climbers—I have seen African black crakes, *Porzana flavirostra*, walking along branches 30 ft. (9 m) above the ground.

By contrast the coots are far more aquatic, and the only members of the Rallidae to have their toes edged with membranous lobes. These increase the surface area of the feet which assists in swimming. Although virtually all of the other rails can swim, they tend not to; but they never venture far from water and the vast majority live in marshy habitats. Many eat invertebrates, insects, nestlings and snails, while others are mostly vegetarian: the purple swamphen, *Porphyrio porphyrio*, is something of a pest in rice-growing areas, as large numbers feed on the shoots of cultivated rice.

Members of Rallidae can be found in the wetlands of every continent, and many species are very common. However, some are not so numerous. The island species (25 percent of which cannot fly) in particular have been taken to the brink by introduced snakes, rats and domestic cats. Captive breeding has helped several rails; and reintroductions have given some cause for optimism for birds that would otherwise be extinct, like the Guam rail, *Rallus owstoni*.

Size

Crakes: 5–10 in. (13–25 cm).
Rails: 5–21 in. (13–53 cm).
Coots: 14–23 in. (35–58 cm).
Gallinules: 10–25 in. (25–63 cm).

Compatibility

Generally speaking, members of the Rallidae up to about 10 in. (25 cm) in length can be kept with other birds of equal size. But some of the larger rails can be very aggressive, especially when they are defending their young; and any other bird of comparable size may be chased, injured or killed. The great majority of the Rallidae also rob nests of eggs and young, and may prey upon fledglings if given the opportunity.

Diet

Diet J (see page 57) for rails.

Management

The Rallidae species have poor to nonexistent flying abilities, but they are often good climbers, and can run up wire mesh—a roofed enclosure is therefore essential. Equally important is plenty of vegetation, especially for newly imported birds which are always very nervous. Tall grass, bushes and reeds should furnish the aviary; and if a shallow pool and running water are provided, the birds will feel considerably more secure.

All of the rail species are fairly hardy and can live outdoors in the summer. But these largely terrestrial birds can suffer from frostbitten toes and must be shut into a frost-free, and preferably heated, house during severe weather. Also, the aviary substrate must be a soft material, such as grass or peat moss, to protect the feet from bumblefoot. (See Ailments—bumblefoot.)

Breeding

Sexing: nearly all monomorphic.

Eggs: 2–16, cream or brown, often with red, brown or black spots or blotches.

Incubation: 18–25 days, normally by both parents.

The breeding aviary does not need to be especially large, but it must have plenty of dense vegetation, including low bushes and tall grasses. A pool and stream are also conducive to breeding, since nests are usually built near or over water. Both sexes normally build the nest, using grasses and reeds to make an open, cup-shaped structure; and some species pull the surrounding vegetation together to form a domed roof.

In captivity, empty plant baskets are sometimes used as nest platforms. Place one near the ground and another about 3 ft. (90 cm) up. Try to position them near water to give the birds a greater feeling of security.

The young are subprecocial, often leaving the nest within hours of hatching. But they cannot feed themselves immediately, and rely on food presented in their parents' bills for the first few days. Thereafter, the chicks follow the adults' example, and start to pick up food themselves; and up to 8 weeks later they are independent.

Chicks are easy to cater for by adding extra mealworms and waxworms to the standard diet. Very finely chopped, hard-boiled egg is also valuable. All of the foods should be as fine as possible to make it easy for the chicks to feed themselves.

Shorebirds

Order: Charadriiformes
Families: Charadriidae (Lapwings and Plovers) 66 species
Recurvirostridae (Avocets and Stilts) 13 species
Burhinidae (Thick-knees) 9 species
Jacanidae (Jacanas) 8 species

Although the shorebirds encompass 12 families, here I have highlighted only the main avicultural ones.

Charadriidae

Lapwings and plovers are short-billed wading birds of cosmopolitan distribution; and are usually black, brown or white. The lapwings often have wing spurs, crests, iridescent plumage and facial wattles or lappets; and sometimes the middle and outer toes are webbed. Plovers tend to be smaller, usually with a black collar and a white nape.

Unlike some of the other shorebirds, lapwings and plovers can only use their short bills to catch visible prey, rather than probing for it beneath the surface of mud or water. Consequently they need fairly open environments, so their food (insects and larvae) can be more easily found and caught. The habitats of these birds are remarkably varied: the southern lapwing, *Vanellus chilensis*, prefers the tropical regions of the South American pasturelands and even urban areas. The crowned plover, *Vanellus coronatus*, can be found throughout Africa in places with very short or burned grass, or semidesert; and the gray plover, *Pluvialis squatarola*, breeds in the high Arctic and migrates to South America, South Africa and Australia for the winter.

Recurvirostridae

This is a small family with an almost worldwide distribution. It comprises 4 avocets (genus *Recurvirostra*), 8 stilts of the genus *Himantopus* and 1 stilt of the genus *Cladorhynchus*. They are long-legged birds, with long bills that are straight in the stilts and upward curved (recurved) in the avocets. The stilts are all similar in appearance; and the 8 *Himantopus* species are so similar to each other, that they are sometimes described as a single species (*H. himantopus*).

Stilts and avocets can be found in fresh, salt or brackish water, in marshes, lagoons and estuaries. They feed on small fish, crustaceans, insects, beetles, flies, dragonflies and brine shrimp. Stilts use their straight bills to strike at prey in deepish water, while the avocets sweep their recurved bills through the water in gentle scything motions. The avocets and the banded stilt have webbed feet and are good swimmers. The *Himantopus* stilts are also capable of swimming, although their feet are only very slightly webbed.

Burhinidae

The thick-knees or stone curlews are generally heavily built, large-eyed, mostly nocturnal birds, with thick ankle joints that can be mistaken for knees. They are highly terrestrial and live in dry habitats, such as on the sand and pebbles of riverbanks, or in country dotted with scrub and low vegetation. Most have short, stout bills that may be used to eat small lizards, frogs, mollusks, rodents, insects and young birds. Thick-knees have a very wide distribution in the tropical and temperate parts of the Eastern Hemisphere; and also in Central and South America.

Jacanidae

Jacanas are rail-like birds with exceptionally long toes and claws, which allow them to run over floating vegetation and lily pads. They also swim well and can even dive beneath the surface. Jacanas can be found in Central and South America, throughout Asia and Australasia, and in Africa where they are often called "lily-trotters." They can be found in almost any tropical or subtropical environment with marshes and rich aquatic vegetation. Their diet includes water weeds and seeds; and a large amount of insects and mollusks, that are found both in the water and on plant leaves.

Size

Charadriidae: 6–16 in. (15–40 cm).

Recurvirostridae: 12–20 in. (30–50 cm).
Burhinidae: 14–21 in. (35–53 cm).
Jacanidae: 8–13 in. (20–33 cm). Not including the long tail of the pheasant-tailed jacana.

Compatibility

Because of their robust build and omnivorous feeding habits, the thick-knees should not be housed with smaller birds. And unlike most of the other shorebirds, they are not gregarious and should only be kept in pairs—occasionally, even this will not work and birds may have to be separated.

Lapwings, plovers, stilts, avocets and jacanas tend to live in pairs or groups, and are usually safe in the company of other birds. However, some species are highly territorial during the breeding season and will need to be given their own aviary.

Diet

Diet K (see page 51). Some of the shorebirds may eat small seeds or grain; but it is not an important part of their diet and I have never found it to be well-liked.

Management

Aviary design: although most shorebirds wade and feed in wet areas, they must also have access to dry ground. The ideal aviary should have well-drained turf, a small patch of clean sand, and a gradually deepening pool fed by running water. The pool is especially important for stilts and avocets, although plovers and lapwings will also use it for paddling, bathing and drinking.

The jacanas need watery areas more than most shorebirds; and the best conditions are provided by a large pool or lake with floating water plants. In captivity, artificial plants and lily pads can create an authentic habitat until the real plants have matured.

The thick-knees are terrestrial birds and do not especially need water, except for normal drinking and bathing purposes.

Hardiness: most of the shorebirds are relatively hardy and can be kept outdoors, with the exception of the jacanas, which do not tolerate the cold very well. I have kept stilts, avocets, plovers and lapwings outside through snow and ice. During wintery evenings they were shut into their heated house; but in the day, they commuted between the shelter and the snow-covered enclosure with no ill-effects. However, the feet of shorebirds may suffer if they are forced to stand on freezing ground for any period of time.

Breeding

Sexing: all monomorphic. However, females of jacanas, plovers and lapwings are often larger than the males.

Eggs and incubation:

Charadriidae: usually 2–4 eggs. Both sexes incubate for 24–28 days.

Recurvirostridae: usually 4 eggs. Both sexes incubate for 22–26 days.

Burhinidae: 1–3 eggs. Both sexes incubate for 25–27 days.

Jacanidae: usually 4 eggs. Only the male incubates for 22–24 days.

Plovers, lapwings, stilts and avocets live in pairs or small flocks; and jacanas sometimes gather in flocks of over 100. But it is only the avocets and stilts that breed in colonies, and of them only the avocets have the best chance of breeding colonially in the aviary. This is because they nest very close together with little or no territoriality, while the stilts will nest up to about 60 ft. (18 m) apart. So for breeding purposes, it is best to keep most shorebird species in pairs within an aviary that is empty of other groundbirds.

In the wild most, if not all, of the jacanas are polyandrous, but in the aviary, polyandry is only likely to be successful in a very large enclosure. In the breeding season the female will take a territory that may encompass those of three or four males. Each male then builds a nest and the female lays a clutch of eggs in each one. The eggs are then incubated solely by the respective male birds.

Jacanas build sparse nests on floating vegetation. But the other shorebirds usually lay their eggs in a simple scrape on the ground, that may or may not be scantily lined with grasses or sticks; and the thick-knees tend to use pebbles, sticks or shells to help disguise the nest.

The chicks of shorebirds are usually highly precocial, being able to run very soon after hatching, although jacanas can take a few days before they are equally mobile. Some jacanas, lapwings and plovers protect their young with "broken-wing" displays, drawing the predator away from the nest by feigning injury. Nearly all species fly overhead uttering their loud, piercing call at the slightest hint of danger, to which the chicks flatten themselves to the ground.

Special foods are not really necessary for the chicks. But they must have plenty of small food items such as finely chopped, hard-boiled egg, and small mealworms, waxworms and crickets. Finely chopped pinkie mice and tiny pieces of meat are also excellent, especially if they are sprinkled with the powdered softbill pellets that feature in diet K. Until the young are a few weeks old, it is a good idea to drain the pool to prevent accidents; and then fill it gradually over a couple of weeks.

Touracos

Order: Cuculiformes
Family: Musophagidae

This family comprises plantain-eaters, go-away birds and touracos, which are all confined to Africa, south of the Sahara. There are 20 species in total, and the name touraco is also often used to describe the plantain-eaters and go-away birds. All are similar in their basic shape, with long tails, short rounded wings and strong feet that are used to run agilely along branches. Nineteen of the species have erectile crests.

The 2 gray plantain-eaters and 3 go-away birds are gray, brown or white; they live in fairly arid, savanna regions, and tend to stay away from closed forest. By contrast, all of the other species (the green touracos and blue plantain-eaters) are birds of the forest and far more beautiful, being green, purple, red or blue. Unique to these birds, are the red and green colors of their feathers: the green is actual pigment and not due to light refraction, while the red contains copper which is soluble in alkaline water.

Most Musophagidae species live in pairs or small groups and are mainly frugivorous, although some will occasionally eat insects. All are sedentary and found at fairly low elevations. But in mountainous regions, such as the Cameroon highlands in West Africa and the Kilimanjaro and Ruwenzori mountains in the east, the following species live at elevations of 6,000–9,000 ft. (1,800–2,700 m): Bannerman's touraco, *Tauraco bannermani*; crested touraco, *T. macrorhynchus*; Ruwenzori touraco, *T. johnstoni*; Hartlaub's touraco, *T. hartlaubi*; and the great blue plantain-eater, *Corythaeola cristata*.

Size

All approximately 15–20 in. (38–50 cm), except the great blue plantain-eater which is 30 in. (75 cm).

Compatibility

Whether a pair of touracos can be kept together, depends greatly on the size of the enclosure. They are territorial birds and in captivity aggression is the main cause of death or injury. The male is generally responsible and even with established pairs constant vigilance is important.

Toward other birds, the touraco species are generally docile and can be kept with smaller, robust softbills such as laughing thrushes. However, during the breeding season these may all be chased by the touracos and have to be removed.

Diet

Frugivore diet C (see page 52). Live food such as mealworms and waxworms can also be offered, although it is largely ignored outside of the breeding season. Touracos swallow their food whole and should be fed fruits that are diced into 1-centimeter cubes. Many species also eat leaves, buds and flowers, especially the gray plantain-eaters and go-away birds. Keep potentially toxic plants out of the aviary, and make use of tough varieties such as conifers.

Management

Touracos are easy to acclimate from the wild and thrive on the standard diet. Initially it is a good idea to include extra fruits in the food until the birds have settled down. In spite of their natural tendencies, I have kept several touracos in one aviary for the duration of their quarantine—single species groups of Hartlaub's and white-cheeked touracos were often quarantined in this way without incident.

In the long term, touracos can be aggressive toward their partners, and benefit from a large aviary. A pair will usually live in an aviary of about 20 ft. x 8 ft. x 8 ft. high (6 m x 2.4 m x 2.4 m). Enclosures two or three times bigger will even accommodate 2 different pairs of touraco species.

Acclimated birds are quite hardy, especially the higher altitude species mentioned above. They can live outside all year, but must have access to a shelter which should be slightly heated during freezing weather. Touracos tend to roost in the outdoor flight and may have to be chased into their house during cold nights or bad weather. To protect them from bumblefoot, perches should be kept clean and replaced periodically.

Breeding

Sexing: all species monomorphic, except the white-bellied go-away bird, *Criniferoides leucogaster*: females may have a greenish beak.

Eggs: green and blue species; usually 2 whitish spherical eggs. Gray species; 2 or 3 blue-tinged eggs.

Incubation: both sexes share incubation which begins with the laying of the first egg.

Green species 18–23 days.
Blue species 24–26 days.
Gray species 26–28 days.

New pairs must be introduced carefully; preferably they should be housed in view of each other, and in adjacent aviaries for 2 weeks. A stress-free introduction can then be affected by using a connecting door. Pairing up birds before they are sexually mature (at one or 2 years of age) may improve the chances of amicability when the breeding cycle begins.

If problems occur, it is usually because the male is aggressive. He is easily capable of killing the female and must be removed immediately if his attentions are severe. Lightly clipping 1 of his wings will give the female an advantage, and perhaps lead to a long-term solution; but sometimes getting a replacement male is the only option.

All of the touraco species tend to build flimsy, pigeonlike nests, with platforms of twigs so thin that the eggs may be visible from beneath. It is therefore important to provide more secure, artificial nest sites. Wire mesh or wooden trays of 12 in. (30 cm) square with 3 in. (8 cm) high sides should be fixed in high, well-concealed locations. Large open-fronted boxes, like fruit boxes, may also be used successfully. Place some thin twigs in the tray or box, and leave plenty on the aviary floor. Both sexes build the nest.

The eggshell and chicks' droppings are usually eaten by the parents. The chicks' eyes open almost immediately after hatching, and at 11 or 12 days of age, young touracos begin to clamber on nearby branches. Some species are aided by a vestigial claw on the bend (alula) of each wing, which disappears as the chicks grow older. This is a vulnerable time for the young birds, since they can easily fall from the nest and die. Provide branches by which they can climb back; or check the aviary regularly so that they can be picked up and returned to the nest by hand.

Both sexes feed the chicks by regurgitation. The preferred rearing foods can vary with the species, but generally fruits and berries are essential; live food and bread or sponge cake moistened in nectar should also be offered. At about 4 weeks of age the chicks leave the nest for good, and 2 to 3 weeks later they are independent. At this stage it is best to remove them because the adult male can become very aggressive.

Fruit Pigeons and Doves

Order: Columbiformes
Family: Columbidae

The terms "pigeon" and "dove" are often used interchangeably, but normally the smaller, more delicate, birds are called doves and the larger ones, called pigeons. The approximately 300 species inhabit most of the world and feed on seeds and fruits. More than 100 of them are softbills, which are broadly described by 3 genera:

Genus *Treron* **(Green Pigeons)**

There are about 23 species, the majority of which are unknown to aviculture. They have strong feet and tend to be sluggish birds, using their predominantly green plumage as the perfect camouflage. The green pigeons are arboreal, living mainly in small groups, and sometimes gathering into huge flocks to feed on fruits and wild figs. Most do not come to the ground except to drink, although some species descend onto crops like maize and rice. Interestingly, the green pigeons are able to grind up hard foods such as seeds and maize, using grit in their gizzard—something the fruit doves and imperial pigeons cannot do. The green pigeons are tropical birds of the forest and secondary growth; and they come from North Africa, India and throughout Southeast Asia, including Japan, Taiwan, Malaysia, Thailand, Indonesia and the Philippines.

Genus *Ducula* **(Imperial Pigeons)**

There are 36 *Ducula* species. Most of them live in small parties that search for food during the day and return to communal roosts at night. They eat fruits and berries but are unable to grind up the seeds: the gizzard is thin and does not contain grit, but instead has numerous horny bumps which strip the flesh from the fruits, leaving the seeds intact; and the intestines of imperial pigeons are particularly short and wide, which allows seeds and nuts to be defecated whole. In this way, such birds act as an important mechanism for dispersing viable seeds throughout the tropics.

Genus *Ptilinopus* (Fruit Doves)

The fruit doves are close relatives of the imperial pigeons, and share the same basic diet and digestive system; but by far their most distinctive feature is their brilliant plumage. The males have bright colors on their heads and underparts that contrast sharply with their green bodies, while the females are often a paler green, and generally far less colorful. Most of the 49 species are found in the Australasian region, with a handful occurring in the Philippines, Malaysia and the nearby Indonesian islands. Fruit doves are arboreal, forest birds, that dislike coming near to the ground unless drawn by food or a potential nest-site; and some, like the jambu, *P. jambu*, are semimigratory, occasionally flying great distances in search of food or roosting places.

Size

Genus *Treron*: 8–14 in. (20–35 cm).
Genus *Ducula*: 15–22 in. (38–55 cm).
Genus *Ptilinopus*: 6–18 in. (15–45 cm) Commonly kept species such as the jambu fruit dove, *P. jambu*, 10 in. (25 cm).

Compatibility

The fruit pigeons and doves are normally very docile and safe with other softbills, although some aggression may occur between pairs during the breeding season. Imperial pigeons, especially, can be aggressive toward each other, and generally most male pigeons and doves will chase the female prior to breeding. But such chases should not cause injury and tend to be restricted to normal breeding behavior.

Diet

Diet C (see page 52) for frugivores, with no additions necessary. Newly purchased birds may be reluctant to feed and should be given a lot of clearly visible berries, diced fruits and peas.

Try not to give the pigeons access to open nectar dishes or very sticky foods, because they will tend to get nectar and fruit pieces stuck to their faces, sometimes forming large lumps. Similar accumulations can form on their feet, eventually causing gangrene and the loss of the foot or toe. (See Ailments—gangrene.)

Management

Newly purchased columbids can be quite scruffy and benefit from a daily spraying with tepid water. Their preen glands are small or nonexistent, and the feathers are cleaned and lubricated by means of special plumes that disintegrate into a powder. Consequently, even established birds thoroughly enjoy being sprayed by a mister system, fine hose or plant sprayer, and will lean over with a wing outstretched to receive the water.

Once acclimated, the green and imperial pigeons are quite hardy, and may live outside year-round. If they are provided with a frost-free shelter, and protected from severe weather, they should not need heat during the winter. The fruit doves, however, do need heated winter accommodation in temperate climates; acclimated birds are otherwise fairly hardy.

Breeding

Sexing: Genus *Treron*. Dimorphic and monomorphic.
Genus *Ducula*. Great majority monomorphic.
Genus *Ptilinopus*. Great majority dimorphic; magnificent (wompoo) fruit dove, *P. magnificus*, monomorphic.
Eggs: Genus *Treron*. Virtually all species, 2 white eggs.
Genus *Ducula*. Probably all species, 1 white egg.
Genus *Ptilinopus*. All species, 1 white egg, mostly with an incubation period of 18 or 19 days.

With a good diet and a suitable environment, fruit doves and pigeons are often willing to breed in captivity. Nests are built in trees and bushes, and I have even seen jambu fruit doves, *P. jambu*, nest on the ground. Frequently the nests are flimsy and in the case of fruit doves can amount to 5 short sticks balanced on a palm frond. Breeding success is therefore much more likely if the birds can be encouraged to use an artificial platform, such as a square, wire-mesh basket.

The platform can be lined with thin twigs to help stimulate

breeding. The adults will then break off more twigs from the surrounding trees (up to 30 m away) and complete the nest themselves. Both sexes usually build the nest and incubate; and there is a general tendency for the female to incubate during the night and early morning. Pigeon chicks grow very fast and are nourished by a "crop milk" which is produced by both sexes. This is the sole source of food for the first few days. As the chick grows, the production of crop milk decreases until the young pigeon is receiving only the adult food.

Young pigeons tend to leave the nest before they can fly properly, and sometimes fall to the floor. The parents ignore them, and such birds quickly become weak and die. It is therefore important to check the aviary regularly so that a fallen chick can be returned to its nest or perch as soon as possible. If the chick appears cold or lethargic, warm it in your hands and wait until it is fully revived before leaving it.

Further Reading (for the species accounts)

Howard, R. and Moore, A. *A Complete Checklist of the Birds of the World.* Second Edition. Academic Press, 1991.

Mobbs, A. J. *Hummingbirds.* Triplegate, 1982.

Rutgers, A. and Norris, K. A. (Editors) *Encyclopedia of Aviculture*, Volumes I to III. Blanford Press, 1977.

Vince, C. *Keeping Softbilled Birds.* Stanley Paul, 1980.

Diet Index

To find the correct diet for your softbill, find your softbill species in this index and note the diet type (Diet A–Diet K) from the list below.
- A. meat-biased omnivore (see page 51)
- B. fruit-biased omnivore (see page 51)
- C. frugivore (see page 52)
- D. hummingbird (see page 52)
- E. sunbird and spiderhunter (see page 53)
- F. other nectivore (see page 53)
- G. standard insectivore (see page 53)
- H. difficult insectivore (see page 54)
- I. carnivore (see page 56)
- J. rail (see page 57)
- K. shorebird (see page 57)

Accentor: 80 percent diet G + 15 percent diced fruits + 5 percent canary seed, all mixed together.
Alethe: Diet G
Ani: Diet A
Antbird: Diet G
Apali: Diet G
Aracari: Diet B
Avocet: Diet K
Babax: Diet A
Babbler:
   scimitar, tit, wren: Diet G
   shrike babbler and most other species: 85 percent Diet G + 15 percent diced fruits in separate dish.
Bananaquit: Diet F
Barbet:
   African and Asian: Diet A
   South American: Diet B
Barwing: Diet A
Bee eater: Diet H
Bellbird: Diet B
Bird of paradise: Diet B
Blackbird: Diet A

Bluethroat: Diet G
Blue robin: Diet G
Bokmakierie: 60 percent diet G + 30 percent diet I + 10 diced fruits, all mixed together.
Boubou: As for bokmakierie.
Broadbill:
   lesser green: Diet B
   long-tailed: Diet G
Bulbul: Diet B
Bushchat: Diet G
Bush robin: Diet G
Bush shrike: 60 percent diet G + 30 percent diet I + 10 percent diced fruits, all mixed together.
Cacique: Diet A
Camaroptera: Diet G
Catbird: Diet A
Chat: Diet G
Chlorophonia: Diet B
Chloropsis: Diet B
Cissa: Diet A
Cisticola: Diet G
Cochoa: 50 percent diet G + 50 per-

cent diced fruits, all mixed together.
Cock-of-the-rock: Diet B
Conebill: Diet G
Coot: Diet J
Cotinga: Diet B
Coucal: 95 percent diet J + 5 percent chopped "fuzzie" mice.
Cowbird: Diet A
Crake: Diet J
Crombec: Diet G
Crow: Diet A
Cuckoo: Diet G
Curlew: Diet K
Cutia: Diet A
Dacnis: Diet F
Dikkop: Diet K
Dotterel: Diet K
Dowitcher: Diet K
Drongo: 85 percent diet G + 15 percent diced fruits in separate dish.
Eremomela: Diet G
Euphonia: Diet B
Fairy bluebird: Diet B
Fiscal shrike: 60 percent diet G + 40 percent diet I, all mixed together.
Flowerpecker: Diet F
Flowerpiercer: Diet F
Forktail: Diet G
Friarbird: Diet B
Frogmouth: 50 percent diet G + 50 percent diet I, all mixed together.
Fruit dove and pigeon: Diet C
Fruitsucker: Diet B
Flycatcher:
  virtually all species: Diet G
  paradise: Diet G/H
  monarch: Diet G/H
  fantail: Diet G/H
  wattle-eye: Diet G/H
  silky (Bombycillidae): Diet A
Fulvetta: Diet G
Gallinule: Diet J

Gnatcatcher/eater: Diet G
Go-away bird: Diet C
Godwit: Diet K
Gonolek: 70 percent diet G + 25 percent diced fruits + 5 percent diet I, all mixed.
Grackle: Diet A
Grandala: 80 percent diet G + 20 percent diced fruits, all mixed together.
Greenbul: Diet B
Greenlet: Diet G
Greenshank: Diet K
Ground hornbill: Diet I
Honeycreeper: Diet F
Honeyeater: Diet B
Hoopoe:
  wood: 90 percent diet G + 10 percent diced fruits in separate dish.
  common *Upupa epops*: Diet G
Hornbill: Diet A + the occasional chopped or whole mouse.
Hummingbird: Diet D
Hunting cissa: Diet A
Iora: Diet B
Ixulus: Diet F
Jacamar: Diet H
Jacana: Diet K
Jay: Diet A
Kingfisher:
  forest species: 60 percent diet G + 40 percent diet I, all mixed together.
  aquatic species: 30 percent diet G + 70 percent diet I, all mixed together.
Kookaburra: Diet I
Knot: Diet K
Lapwing: Diet K
Leafbird: Diet B
Liocichla: Diet A
Longclaw: Diet G
Magpie: Diet A

Magpie robin: Diet G
Manakin: Diet B
Marshbird: Diet A
Meadowlark: 85 percent diet A + 15 percent canary seed, all mixed together.
Minla: Diet A
Minivet: Diet G
Mockingbird: Diet A
Monarch (flycatcher): Diet G/H
Moorhen: Diet J
Motmot: 80 percent diet G + 20 percent diced fruits in separate dish.
Mousebird: Diet C
Mynah: Diet A
Nicator: 60 percent diet G + 30 percent diet I + 10 percent chopped fruits, all mixed together.
Nighthawk: Diet G
Nightjar: Diet G
Niltava: Diet G
Nuthatch: Diet G
Orangequit: Diet F
Oriole (Old World and New World): Diet A
Oropendola: Diet A
Ovenbird: 80 percent diet G + 20 percent diet I, all mixed together.
Oxpecker: Diet G
Oystercatcher: Diet K
Parrotbill: 65 percent diet G + 35 percent diced fruits, all mixed together.
Pekin robin: Diet A
Phalarope: Diet K
Piculet: 75 percent diet G + 25 percent diced fruits, all mixed together.
Piha: Diet B
Pipit: Diet G
Pitta: Diet G
Plantain-eater: Diet C
Plover: Diet K

Pratincole: Diet K
Prinia: Diet G
Rail: Diet J
Red-billed leiothrix: Diet A
Redshank: Diet K
Redstart: Diet G
Roadrunner: Diet I
Robin: Diet G
Robin chat: Diet G
Roller: Diet G/H + the occasional small mouse, lizard or frog.
Rubythroat: Diet G
Sandpiper: Diet K
Sandplover: Diet K
Saw-wing: Diet G
Shama: Diet G
Shortwing: Diet G
Shrike:
  cuckoo: Diet G
  gonolek: 70 percent diet G + 25 percent diced fruits + 5 percent diet I, all mixed together.
  most other species: 60 percent diet G + 30 percent diet I + 10 percent chopped fruits, all mixed together.
Sibia: Diet A
Silky flycatcher (*Bombycillidae*): Diet A
Silver-eared mesia: Diet A
Siva: Diet A
Snipe: Diet K
Spiderhunter: Diet E
Starling:
  most species: Diet A
  amethyst (or violet); and the genera *Lamprotornis* and *Cosmopsarus*: 75 percent diet G + 25 percent diced fruits, fed in separate dishes.
Stilt: Diet K
Stint: Diet K
Stonechat: Diet G
Sugarbird (honeycreepers): Diet F
Sunbird: Diet E

Sunbittern: Diet J
Tailorbird: Diet G
Tanager:
  most tanagers: Diet B
  ant: 90 percent diet G + 10 percent diced fruits in separate dish.
  chlorochrysa: 90 percent diet G + 10 percent diced fruits in separate dish.
  chlorophonia: Diet B
  conebill: Diet G
  euphonia: Diet B
  shrike: 80 percent diet G + 20 percent diced fruits in separate dish.
  swallow: Diet G
  Dacnis, flowerpiercer, honeycreeper and orangequit: Diet F
Tattler: Diet K
Tesia: Diet G
Thick-knee: Diet K
Thrasher: Diet A
Thrush:
  ground: 70 percent diet G + 30 percent diced fruits in separate dish.
  laughing: Diet A
  most other species: 50 percent diet G + 50 percent diced fruits in separate dish.
Tit: Diet G
Toucan, toucanet and aracari: Diet B
Touraco: Diet C
Treecreeper: Diet G
Tree pie: Diet A
Trembler: Diet A
Trogon:
  South American: 65 percent diet G + 35 percent diced fruits in separate dish.
  Asian: 80 percent diet H + 20 percent diced fruits in separate dish.
  African: 80 percent diet H + 20 percent diced fruits in separate dish.
Troupial: Diet A
Turnstone: Diet K
Tyrant: Diet G
Umbrellabird: Diet B
Vireo: 85 percent diet G + 15 percent diced fruits in separate dish.
Wagtail: Diet G
Wallcreeper: Diet G
Warbler: 90 percent diet G + 10 percent finely diced fruits in separate dish.
Water hen: Diet J
Wattle-eye: Diet G
Waxwing: Diet C
Whistler: Diet G
White eye: Diet F
Wren: Diet G
Woodcock: Diet K
Wood hoopoe: 90 percent diet G + 10 percent diced fruits in separate dish.
Woodpecker: 80 percent diet G + 20 percent diced fruits in separate dish.
Yellowthroat: Diet G
Yuhina: Diet F
Zosterop: Diet F

Index
Common and Scientific Names

In the following listing, italicized numbers refer to pictures.

A

Abyssinian ground hornbill 88
Aceros plicatus subruficollis 159
Acridotheres albocinctus 151
A. tristis 218
African black crake *135, 176,* 252
African glossy starling 220
African spur-winged plover *171*
African trogon 54
Alcedo cristata 156
American robin 79
Amethyst starling 219
Anchieta's sunbird 201
Andean cock-of-the-rock *132*
Anisognathus flavinuchus 178
Anthracoceros malabaricus 158
Apteryx australis mantelli 91
Aracari 91, 127, 241, 243
Asian fairy bluebird *146,* 190, 191
Asian pied starling *150*
Asian trogon 54
Aulacorhynchus prasinus 168
Australian bee eater 229
Avocet 57, 91, 128, 255, 257
Azure-winged magpie 222

B

Babbler 15, 79, 185
Baillonius bailloni 166
Bali mynah 88, *149*
Bananaquit 53
Band-tailed oropendola 225
Banded pitta *148,* 207
Bannerman's touraco 260

Barbet 15, 50, 51, 80, 82, 91, 120, 128, 245, 246
Basilornis celebensis 40, *134, 149,* 219
Bay-headed tanager *141*
Bearded reedling 79, *130, 132*
Bee hummingbird 248
Bee eater 50, 54, 61, 81, 127, 228
Berenicornis comatus 159
Bird of paradise 51
Black-headed gonolek *132*
Black-headed woodpecker *130*
Black-knobbed imperial pigeon *173*
Black-mantled fairy bluebird 191
Black-naped fruit dove 88, *130, 174*
Black-necked aracari *129, 166*
Blue and yellow tanager *129, 139,* 179
Blue magpie 222
Blue-bearded bee eater 229
Blue-cheeked bee eater 228
Blue-gray tanager 15, 88, *140,* 178, 179
Blue-necked tanager *141*
Blue-winged kookaburra 238, 240
Blue-winged mountain tanager 178
Blue-winged pitta 207
Bluethroat 53
Blyth's hornbill *159*
Brazilian tanager 178
Broadbill 15, 127, 209, 212, 213, 214
Brown bulbul 215
Brown kiwi 91
Brown-breasted barbet *163*
Buceros bicornis 88, *158, 159,* 234
B. hydrocorax 88

272

B. rhinoceros 88, *159*
Bucorvus abyssinicus 88
Bulbul 47, 51, 127, 215, 216
Burhinos capensis 170
Bush robin 53

C

Calypte costae 169
C. helenae 248
Calyptomena 212
C. viridis 142, 212
Cape thick-knee *170*
Carmine bee eater 228
Chat 15, 53, 119
Chestnut-flanked white eye 196
Chestnut-mandibled toucan *165*
Chlorocharis emilae 196
Chlorophanes spiza 183
Chlorophonia 51, 127, 177, 180, 181
Chloropsis 15, 51, 79, 80, 127, *144*, 193, 194, 195, 213
C. aurifrons 194
C. a. media 194
C. hardwickei 145
C. sonnerati 144, 195
Cinnamon white eye 196
Cinnyricinclus leucogaster 219
Cissilopha jay 222
Cissilopha sanblasiana 138
Cock-of-the-rock 81, 91
Colibri coruscans 250
Colius striatus 133
Columba guinea phaenota 117
Coot 57, 128
Coppersmith barbet 246
Copsychus malabaricus 154, 203
C. saularis 154, 203
Coracias benghalensis 232
C. caudata 88, *161*, 232
C. garrulus 232
C. spatulata *161*, 232
Corythaeola cristata 260
Cosmopsarus regius 219, 221
Costa's hummingbird *169*

Cotinga 51
Crake 57, 128
Crested oropendola 225, 226
Crested touraco 260
Criniferoides leucogaster 262
Crow 51, 79, 91, 127, 222
Crowned plover 255
Cuckoo 53, 81
Curlew 57
Cyanerpes caeruleus 183
C. cyaneus 143, *183*
C. lucidus 183
C. nitidus 183
Cyanocorax mystacalis 134, *137*
C. yncas 138
Cyanopica cyana 222
Cyanoptila cyanomelaena 209

D

Dacelo leachii 238
D. novaguineae 88, *157*, 238
Dacnis 53, 177, 178
Dhyal thrush 127, *154*, 203
Diademed tanager *141*
Dotterel 57
Dowitchers 57
Drongo 15, 51
Ducula 264, 265
D. aenea paulina 172
D. myristicivora 173
D. rufigaster 172

E

Elliot's laughing thrush *153*
Emerald glossy starling *149*
Emerald toucanet *168*
Eubucco bourcierii 164, 246
Euphonia 15, 51, 127, 177, 180, 181
Euphonia laniirostris 142
European bee eater 228, 232
Eurypyga helias 88

F

Fairy bluebird 51, 79, 80, 88, 91, 127, 190, 191

Fantail 54
Fire-tufted barbet *164*
Flame-headed barbet *164*, 246
Flowerpiercer 177
Flycatcher 15, 53, 79, 80
Forest kingfisher 238, 239
Frogmouth 99
Fruit dove 38, 51, 79, 83, 91, 103, 128, *172*, 213, 264, 265, 266
Fruit pigeon 15, 38, 51, 79, 83, 103, 128, *172*, 264, 265, 266, 267
Fulvetta 79

G

Gallinule 57, 91, 128
Garrulax 188
G. canorus 188
G. elliotii 153
G. formosus 188
G. galbanus 152, 188
G. leucolophus 153, 188
G. milnei 188
G. pectoralis 188
G. poecilorhynchus 130, 152
Giant barbet 245
Giant hummingbird 248
Giant kingfisher 88
Giant pitta 207
Go-away bird 260
Godwit 57
Golden bush robin *132*
Golden-breasted mynah *150*
Golden-fronted leafbird 194
Grackle 218
Gracula religiosa 120
Gray plover 255
Gray-breasted spiderhunters 200
Gray-headed kingfisher *155*
Great blue plantain-eater 260
Great Indian hornbill 88, *158, 160*
Greater necklaced thrush 188
Greater niltava *147*
Green aracari *165*
Green honeycreeper 183

Green jay *138*
Green magpie 222
Green pigeons 264
Green sunbird 201
Greenbul 215
Grosbeak starling *129*, 220
Ground hornbill 234, 235, 236
Ground thrush 213
Guam kingfisher 88, *155*
Guam rail 88, *176*, 252
Gurney's pitta 207

H

Halcyon chloris 135, 157
H. cinnamomina cinnamomina 88, *155*
H. leucocephala 155
Hardwicke's chloropsis *145*
Hartlaub's touraco 260
Hill mynah 120
Himantopus 256
Hoami thrush 188
Honeycreeper 15, 53, 127, 177, 183
Honeyeater 15, 51
Hooded pita *148,* 207
Hoopoe 53
Hornbill 15, 50, 56, 76, 80, 81, 82, 127, 234
Hummingbird 15, 52, 81, 128, 248, 249, 250
Hunting cissa 222
Hypocryptadius cinnamomeus 196

I

Imperial pigeon 264
Indian hornbill 234
Indian or Oriental white eye 196
Indian roller *161*, 232
Iora 51
Irena cyanogaster 191
I. c. cyanogaster 191
I. c. ellae 191
I. c. hoogstraali 191
I. c. melanochlamys 191

I. puella 88, *146*, 190, 191

J

Jacana 57, 128, 255, 257
Jackson's hornbill *160*
Jambu fruit dove 88, *129*, *173*, 265
Japanese blue flycatcher 209
Japanese white eye 196
Jay 15, 50, 51, 76, 83, 91, 127, 222

K

Kea 117
Kingfisher 50, 56, 61, 81, 91, 127, 238, 239, 240
Kiskadee 15
Knot 57
Kookaburra 56, 91, 127, 238, 239, 240

L

Lamprotornis iris 149
L. superbus 221
Laniarius erythrogaster 132
Lapwing 57, 128, 255, 257
Laughing kookaburra 88, *157*, 238
Laughing thrush 51, 79, 91, 127, 185, 188
Leiothrix argentauris 151, 185, 186
L. lutea 13, 73, *151*, 185, 186, 193
Lesser green broadbill 51, *142*, 213
Leucospar rothschildi 88, *149*
Levaillant's barbet *163*
Lilac-breasted roller 88, *161*, 232
Liocichla 185
Liocichla phoenicea 132
L. steerii 193
Livingstone's touraco *174*
Long-tailed broadbill 212, 213
Lybius melanopterus 163

M

Magnificent (wompoo) fruit dove 266
Magpie 15, 50, 51, 75, 83, 91, 127, 203, 222
Malachite kingfisher *156*

Manakin 15, 51
Marianas fruit dove 88
Marshbird 51
Masked plover *171*
Megaceryle torquata 88
Megalaima haemacephala 246
M. virens 245
Merops albicollis 163, 228
M. apiaster 228
M. nubicus 228
M. ornatus 229
M. superciliosus 228
Mesia 79, 80
Minivets 53
Minla 79
Mino dumontii 150
Mockingbird 51
Monarch flycatchers 54
Montezuma oropendola *136,* 225
Motmot 15
Mount Omei liocichlas 80
Mountain tanager 15
Mouse-colored sunbird 201
Mousebird 52
Muscicapa thalassina 147, 209
Musophaga violacea 88, *175*
Mynah 51, 80, 91, 127, 217, 218, 219

N

Nectarinia famosa 200
N. jugularis frenata 199
N. olivacea 201
N. seimundi 201
N. veroxii 201
Nestor notabilis 117
Nightjar 99
Niltava 53, 80, 209, 210, 211
N. grandis 147
Northern pied hornbill *158*
Nuthatch 47, 53, 80
Nyctyornis amicta 229, 230
N. athertoni 229

O

Old World flycatchers 127, 209
Olive-backed sunbird 199, 201
Olive-black eye 196
Orangequit 177
Oropendola 51, 127, 225, 226
Owlet-nightjar 99
Oxpecker 217, 218, 219
Oystercatcher 57

P

Pagoda starling 221
Palm tanager 178
Panurus biarmicus 130, *132*
Paradise flycatcher 54, 209
Paradise tanager *140*
Parrot 39
Parrotbill 53
Patagona gigas 248
Pekin robin 13, 51, 73, 79, 80, 91, 127, *151*, 185, 186, 193, 213, 241
Pericrocotus flammeus 132
Phalarope 57
Picus erythropygius 130
Pied barbet 246
Pink-spotted fruit dove 117, *174*
Pitta 15, 53, 119, 127, *148*, 206, 207
Pitta brachyura 207
P. caerulea 207
P. guajana 207
P. gurneyi 207
P. sordida 207
Plantain-eaters 260
Plover 57, 91, 128, 255
Pluvialis squatarola 255
Podargus strigoides 88
Porphyrio porphyrio 176, 252
Porzana flavirostra 135, 176, 252
Psarisomus dalhousiae 212
Psarocoliius latirostris 225
P. decumanus insularis 225, 226
P. montezuma 136, 225
Psilopogon pyrolophus 164

Pterglossus viridis 165
Pteroglossus aracari 129, 166
Ptilinopus 265, 266
P. jambu 88, 129, *173*, 265, 266
P. magnificus 266
P. melanospila 88, *130, 174*
P. perlatus 117, *174*
P. porphyrea 88
P. roseicapillus 88
Puffback flycatcher 209
Purple honeycreeper 183
Purple swamphen *176*, 252
Pycnonotus cafer 148, 216
P. goiavier 216
P. jocosus 215
P. leucogenys 216

Q

Quetzal 120

R

Racquet-tailed roller *161*, 232
Rail 57, 91, 128, 252
Rallus owstoni 88, *176*, 252
Ramphastos swainsonii 165
R. toco 88, *168*, 241
R. tucanus 166
R. vitellinus 241
Ramphocelus bresilius 178
R. carbo 88, *139*, 178
Red and yellow barbet 246
Red-bearded bee eater 229, 230
Red-billed blue magpie *137*
Red-billed hornbill *158*, 234
Red-billed toucan *166*
Red-crested touraco *175*
Red-faced liocichla *132*
Red-legged honeycreeper 183
Red-tailed thrush 188
Red-vented bulbul *149*, 216
Red-whiskered bulbul 215, 216
Red-winged thrush 188
Redshank 57
Redstart 15, 53, 80

Rhinoceros hornbill 88, *159*
Roadrunner 56
Robin 53, 119
Roller 127, 232
Rose-colored starling 219, 221
Royal starling 219, 221
Rubythroat 53
Rufous hornbill 88
Rufous hummingbird 248
Rufous laughing thrush *130*, *152*
Rufous-bellied imperial pigeon *172*
Rupicola peruviana *132*
Ruwenzori touraco 260

S

Saffron toucanet *166*
San-blas jay *138*
Sandpiper 57
Sandplover 57
Sayaca tanager 178
Scarlet minivet *132*, *133*
Schalow's touraco *175*
Scissirostrum dubium *129*, 220
Selasphorus rufus 248
Shama 53, 80, 127
Shining honeycreeper 183
Shorebird 255, 256, 257, 258, 259
Short-billed honeycreeper 183
Shrike 15, 50, 82, 83, 91
Sibia 15, 79
Silver-beaked tanager 88, *139*, 179
Silver-eared mesia 15, 51, 91, 127, *151*, 185, 186, 241
Siva 51
Snipe 57
Southern lapwing 255
Southern speckled pigeons 117
Sparkling violet-eared hummingbird 250
Speckled mousebird *133*
Spiderhunter 15, 47, 53, 127, 199, 200, 201
Starling 15, 50, 51, 75, 80, 91, 127, 217, 218, 219, 220, 221

Steere's liocichla 193
Stephanophorus diadematus *141*
Stilt 57, 127, 241, 255, 257
Stint 57
Sturnus contra 150
S. pagodarum 221
S. roseus 219, 221
S. vulgaris 217
Sulawesi green imperial pigeon *172*
Sulawesi king starling 40, 134, 149, 219
Sunbird 15, 53, 127, 199, 200, 201
Sunbittern 88, 91
Superb starling 221

T

Tanager 15, 47, 51, 76, 79, 80, 91, 120, 127, 177, 180
Tangara chilensis *140*
T. cyanicollis *141*
T. gyrola *141*
T. mexicana 88
Tarsiger chrysaeus *132*
Tauraco marorhynchus 260
T. bannermani 260
T. erythrolophus *175*
T. hartlaubi 260
T. johnstoni 260
T. livingstonii *174*
T. persa schalowi *175*
Tawney frogmouth 88, 91
Temminck's fruit dove 88
Thick-billed euphonias *142*
Thick-knee 127, 255, 257
Thraupis 178
T. bonariensis *129*, *139*
T. episcopus 88, *140*, 178
Thrush 15, 91, 206
Tickbird 217
Tinkerbird 245
Tit 15, 47, 53, 80, 209
Tit babbler 53
Tockus erythrorhynchus *158*, 234
T. flavirostris 234

T. jacksoni 160
Toco toucan 88, *168*, 241
Toucan 39, 50, 51, 82, 91, 120, 128, 241, 242, 243, 244
Toucanet 128, 241
Touraco 38, 51, 52, 79, 81, 91, 120, 128, 260
Trachyphonus erythrocephalus 246
T. vaillantii 163
Treecreeper 53
Treepie 51, 222
Treron 264, 265
Tricholaema leucomelaina 246
Troupial 51, 75
Turdus migratorius 79
Turquoise tanager 88
Tyrant flycatcher 209

U

Urocissa erythrorhyncha 137

V

Vanellus chilensis 255
V. coronatus 255
V. miles 171
Verditer flycatcher *147*, 209
Violaceous plantain-eater *175*
Violet starling 219
Violet touraco 88

W

Wagtail 53, 119
Wallcreeper 53
Warbler 53
Water hen 57

Wattle-eye flycatcher 54, 209
Waxwings 52
White eye 15, 53, 79, 127, 196
White-bellied go-away bird 262
White-cheeked bulbul 216
White-collared kingfisher *135, 157*
White-collared mynah *151*
White-crested laughing thrush *153*, 188
White-crowned hornbill *159*
White-rumped shama thrush *154*, 203
White-tailed jay *134*, *135*, *137*
White-throated bee eater *163*, 228
Woodcock 57
Woodpecker 15, 53, 80, 91
Woodpecker starling 220
Wren 53
Wren babbler 53

Y

Yellow-billed hornbill 234
Yellow-faced mynah *150*
Yellow-spectacled white eye 196
Yellow-throated laughing thrush *152*
Yellow-tufted malachite sunbirds 200
Yellow-vented bulbul 216
Yuhina 15, 53, 79, 91, 185

Z

Zosterops 196
Z. japonica 196
Z. mayottensis 196
Z. palpebrosa 196
Z. wallacei 196

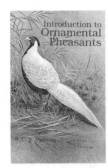

Introduction to Ornamental Pheasants
Keith Howman
5 ½ x 8 ½, HC, 128 pp.
30 color shots & over 40 b/w
ISBN 0-88839-381-4

Natural History of the Waterfowl
Frank S. Todd
10 ½ x 13, HC, 500 pp.
750 color photos
ISBN 0-934797-11-0

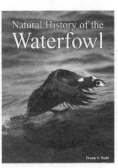

The keeping of ornamental pheasants has grown considerably in recent years and with it the need for a basic, yet comprehensive, book on the subject to guide newcomers through the many aspects of selection and management of these birds.

More than 750 beautifully reproduced photographs of waterfowl in their natural habitat: the most complete photographic presentation of the waterfowl ever published. Frank S. Todd is perhaps best known for his achievements as creator and curator of the largest and most comprehensive collection of waterfowl in North America.

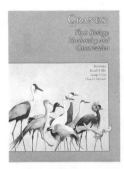

Cranes
Their Biology, Husbandry, and Conservation
Editors: David H. Ellis, George F. Gee and Claire M. Mirande
8 ½ x 11, HC, 336 pp., 16 pp. of color
ISBN 0-88839-385-7

Waterfowl
Care, Breeding and Conservation
Simon Tarsnane
5 ½ x 8 ½, SC, 272 pp.
32 pages of color
0-88839-391-1

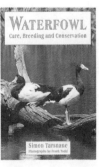

Written by 21 of the world's foremost experts, *Cranes* is the culmination of 25 years of research on these magnificent creatures. Offering a magnificent compendium of crane biology, husbandry and conservation, the book is the most comprehensive and up-to-date tome on cranes, particularly on how to raise them.

Simon Tarsnane has created the ultimate resource for anyone interested in the propagation and preservation of waterfowl. A practical working handbook for both the beginner and the advanced aviculturist, Tarsnane draws on more than 20 years of experience to offer concise and informative data about *all* the waterfowl of the world.

Order From: Hancock Wildlife Research Center
Order Desk: (800) 938-1114 fax: (800) 983-2262
(604) 538-1114 fax: (604) 538-2262
email: hancock@uniserve.com

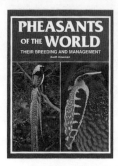

Pheasants of the World
Keith Howman
8 ½ x 11, HC, 184 pp.
340 magnificent color photos plus many drawings
ISBN 0-88839-280-X

Practical Incubation
Rob Harvey
5 ½ x 8 ½, SC, 160 pp.
Over 35 color & 110 b/w photos
ISBN 0-88839-310-5

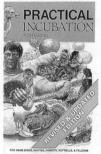

Keith Howman is one of the world's most successful rare pheasant breeders, and as Director General of the World Pheasant Association, he has traveled the world championing the pheasant's cause.

More than 340 spectacular color photographs feature the life works of Jean Howman, Kenneth W. Fink and many others who submitted over 8,000 shots.

Practical Incubation covers all the basics and the finer points: how to control humidity, plot the 15 percent weight loss, even how to deal with partially incubated eggs. This is an indispensable tool for rearing game birds, parrots, falcons and other bird breeds.

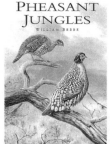

Commercial and Ornamental Game Bird Breeders Handbook
5 ½ x 8 ½, SC, 496 pp.
Over 75 photos & illus.
ISBN 0-88839-311-3

Pheasant Jungles
William Beebe
6 x 9, HC, 246 pp.
ISBN 0-906864-05-4

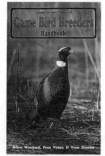

- Includes 8 new color plates by Timothy Greenwood
- Black & white photos throughout

Pheasant Jungles captures the excitement of the solitary pursuit of the scarce and secretive pheasants. A birding classic reprinted.

A. Woodward, P. Vohra & V. Denton

Three of the most imminent researchers in the keeping, rearing and nutritional studies of pheasant, quail and partridge have combined their sixty years of experience to produce this bible of aviculture.

Order From:

Hancock Wildlife Research Center
Order Desk: (800) 938-1114 fax: (800) 983-2262
(604) 538-1114 fax: (604) 538-2262
email: hancock@uniserve.com